# PLAGUE AND THE CITY

*Plague and the City* uncovers discourses of plague and anti-plague measures in the city during the medieval, early modern and modern periods, and explores the connection between plague and urban environments including attempts by professional bodies to prevent or limit the outbreak of epidemic disease.

Bringing together leading scholars of plague, this book provides an inter-disciplinary study of plague in the city across time and space. The chapters cover a wide range of periods, geographical locations and disciplinary approaches but all seek to answer significant questions, including whether common motives can be identified, and how far knowledge about plague was based on an understanding of the urban space. It also examines how maps and photographs contribute to understanding plague in the city through exploring the ways in which the relationship between plague and the urban environment has been visualised, from the poisoned darts of plague winging their way towards their victims in the votive pictures from the Renaissance, to the mapping of the spread of disease in late nineteenth-century Bombay and photographing Honolulu's great plague fire in 1900.

Containing a series of studies that illuminate plague's urban connection as a key social and political concern throughout history, *Plague and the City* is ideal for students of early modern history, and of the early modern city and plague more specifically.

**Lukas Engelmann** is Chancellor's Fellow for Sociology and History of Biomedicine at the University of Edinburgh. His doctoral research focused on the visual medical history of AIDS/HIV. His current research focuses on the digital transformation of epidemiology and the history of epidemiological models and concepts in the long twentieth century.

**John Henderson** is Professor of Italian Renaissance History in the Department of History, Classics and Archaeology, Birkbeck, University of London; Fellow of Wolfson College, University of Cambridge; and Research Professor, Monash University, Melbourne. His previous publications include *The Renaissance Hospital* (2006).

**Christos Lynteris** is Senior Lecturer in Social Anthropology at the University of St Andrews and Principal Investigator of the European Research Council funded research project Visual Representations of the Third Plague Pandemic (2013–2018). His work focuses on the anthropological and historical examination of infectious disease epidemics. His previous books include *The Spirit of Selflessness in Maoist China* (2012), *Ethnographic Plague* (2016), and *Histories of Post-Modern Contagion* (edited with Nicholas Evans, 2018).

# THE BODY IN THE CITY

This series aims to intersect and to energise two strands in historical studies: the pre-modern city as an historical subject (encompassing political institutions, rituals, built environments, religious activities, etc.) and histories of the pre-modern body with their debates about how bodies are shaped by discourse and context. The series will highlight approaches which emphasize the vernacular as revealed by new sources and novel approaches to them. While there are numerous studies of the body in history, this series will explore critically and in innovative ways the relationship between bodies and environments. This will allow scholars involved to analyse how particular spaces, locations and physical *milieux* affect understandings of the body and govern responses to particular problems. The multi-disciplinary approach to the topic places the series at the leading edge of its field.

**Series Editors:** *Peter Howard, Monash University, Australia, and John Henderson, Birkbeck, University of London, UK, and Monash University, Australia*

**In this series:**

**Plague and the City**
*Edited by Lukas Engelmann, John Henderson, and Christos Lynteris*

For more information about this series, please visit: https://www.routledge.com/The-Body-in-the-City/book-series/BOCY

# PLAGUE AND THE CITY

*Edited by*
*Lukas Engelmann, John Henderson,*
*and Christos Lynteris*

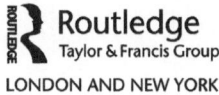

Routledge
Taylor & Francis Group

LONDON AND NEW YORK

First published 2019
by Routledge
2 Park Square, Milton Park, Abingdon, Oxon OX14 4RN

and by Routledge
711 Third Avenue, New York, NY 10017

*Routledge is an imprint of the Taylor & Francis Group, an informa business*

*British Library Cataloguing in Publication Data*
A catalogue record for this book is available from the British Library

*Library of Congress Cataloging in Publication Data*
Names: Engelmann, Lukas, 1981- editor. | Henderson, John, 1949
    June 12- editor. | Lynteris, Christos, editor.
Title: Plague and the city / edited by Lukas Engelmann, John
    Henderson and Christos Lynteris.
Description: Abingdon, Oxon ; New York, NY : Routledge, 2018. |
    Series: The body in the city | Includes bibliographical references.
Identifiers: LCCN 2018028399|
Subjects: LCSH: Plague—History. | Plague—Prevention. | Public
    health History.
Classification: LCC RA644.P7 P385 2018 | DDC 614.5/732—dc23
LC record available at https://lccn.loc.gov/2018028399

ISBN: 978-1-138-59067-0 (hbk)
ISBN: 978-1-138-32612-5 (pbk)
ISBN: 978-0-429-45004-4 (ebk)

Typeset in Bembo
by Swales & Willis Ltd, Exeter, Devon, UK

# CONTENTS

# FIGURES

# PREFACE AND ACKNOWLEDGEMENTS

*Plague and the City* is an output of the Visual Representations of the Third Plague Pandemic project (PI Christos Lynteris) which was funded by a European Research Council Starting Grant under the European Union's Seventh Framework Programme/ERC grant agreement no. 336564. The volume derives from a collection of papers presented at the first annual conference of Visual Representations of the Third Plague Pandemic, which was held at the University of Cambridge's Centre for Research in the Arts, Social Sciences and Humanities (CRASSH) between 5 and 6 December 2014 on the topic of 'Plague and the City: Disease, Epidemic Control, and the Urban Environment'. We would like to thank the conference's participants, Maria Antonia Almeida, Liora Bigon, Carlo Caduff, Neil Cummins, Samuel Cohn, Romola Davenport, Diego Ramiro Farinas, Marta Hanson, Andrea Janku, Pavla Jirkova, and Annamaria Motrescu-Mayes, for their input in the discussion of the relation between plague and the city, and, Emma Hacking, for her wonderful support in organising the conference. The series 'The Body in the City', and this volume, has been made possible by the Monash Faculty of Arts Focus Research Program: 'Body in the City, 1100–1800'.

# CONTRIBUTORS

**Lukas Engelmann** is a Chancellor's Fellow for Sociology and History of Biomedicine at the University of Edinburgh. His doctoral research focused on the visual medical history of AIDS/HIV, which will be published as *Mapping AIDS* in autumn 2018. His current research focuses on the digital transformation of epidemiology and the history of epidemiological models and concepts in the long twentieth century.

**Nicholas H. A. Evans** is a Fellow in the Department of Anthropology at the London School of Economics. His work focuses on understanding the comparative and historical nature of doubt and uncertainty. For his PhD (2014) he carried out ethnographic fieldwork in India, and he has written about religion and ritual in the subcontinent.

**Vanessa Harding** is Professor of London History at Birkbeck, University of London. She has published on population, health, mortality, and burial in early modern London, including a major comparative study of burial in Paris and London, 1500–1670, and more widely on families, housing, and the urban environment.

**John Henderson** is Professor of Italian Renaissance History in the Department of History, Classics and Archaeology, Birkbeck, University of London; Fellow of Wolfson College, University of Cambridge; and Research Professor, Monash University, Melbourne. His previous publications include *The Renaissance Hospital* (2006).

**Christos Lynteris** is Senior Lecturer in Social Anthropology at the University of St Andrews and Principal Investigator of the European Research Council funded research project Visual Representations of the Third Plague Pandemic (2013–2018). His work focuses on the anthropological and historical examination of infectious disease epidemics. His previous books include *The Spirit of Selflessness in Maoist China* (2012), *Ethnographic Plague* (2016), and *Histories of Post-Modern Contagion* (edited with Nicholas Evans, 2018).

**Robert Peckham** is Professor of History and Director of the Centre for the Humanities and Medicine at the University of Hong Kong. He has written widely on histories of medicine, health, and disease in colonial and postcolonial Asia. Recent publications include the book *Epidemics in Modern Asia* (2016) and the edited volume *Empires of Panic: Epidemics and Colonial Anxieties* (2015).

**Branwyn Poleykett** is a Research Fellow at the Wellcome Centre for Cultures and Environments of Health at the University of Exeter. She is currently writing a book on health communication in Senegal.

**Carole Rawcliffe** is Professor Emerita of Medieval History at the University of East Anglia. She has published widely on medical practice, disease (especially leprosy), the history of hospitals and ideas about personal and public health in the later Middle Ages, with a particular emphasis on the English urban environment.

# INTRODUCTION

## The plague and the city in history

*Lukas Engelmann, John Henderson, and
Christos Lynteris*

Plague, like many epidemic diseases, has long been associated with the city. Aspects of urban life, like population density, squalor, and poverty, immoral behaviour, and civil unrest, have been invoked in explaining plague outbreaks. This convergence rests as much on the long history of imagining urban space as prone to disease and illness, as on the projection of an image of plague as a disease driven ultimately by human settlement.

This volume explores the way in which plague and the city have become connected in a range of epidemic narratives, epidemiological perspectives, and anti-epidemic interventions. Key to this endeavour is the examination of how governments or professional bodies across the centuries have sought to adopt measures first to prevent plague outbreaks in urban terrains and then to mitigate their effect once, despite their best intentions, they had broken out. This theme is furthermore explored through the many ways in which plague in the city was imagined and visualised, from the poisoned darts of plague winging their way towards their victims in the votive pictures of the Renaissance, to the mapping of the spread of disease in the late nineteenth and early twentieth century in Bombay or French Morocco to the photographic record of anti-plague operations in Hong Kong and Honolulu.

The contributions to this volume trace the visual and written representation of plague as a disease in and of the urban environment across periods and regions in the historical past. In doing so, this collection will seek to underline the trans-historical affinity of themes, tropes, and images across the centuries. Through the combination of different perspectives and case studies, the volume seeks to clarify how common motifs of poverty, stench, housing, and dirt have shaped the urban character of plague. The volume also contributes to the historiography of urban space and asks to what extent it has been discovered, mapped, and understood through images, maps, and photographs of plague.

## Urban pathologies

Over fourteen centuries and three pandemics, from the devastation of Constantinople in 542, Giovanni Boccaccio's Black Death in Florence in 1348, the Great Plague of London in 1665, and the Moscow plague riots of 1771 to the torching of Honolulu's Chinatown in 1900 and the inter-imperial struggle over plague-stricken Harbin in 1911, the disease has given shape to numerous urban crises and to visions of a new, plague-free urban future. Arising from diverse theories and interpretations of the disease, measures to combat plague focused on urban and housing forms, as well as particularly 'urban' living habits, which were seen as catalysts in the transmission and persistence of plague.

The association between disease, dirt, and the urban environment has a long pedigree, whether in historical terms in relation to Imperial Roman sanitation and urban planning or in relation to the historical and anthropological tradition inspired by Mary Douglas's seminal work on *Purity and Danger*.[1]

This volume, however, begins with the middle ages when urban centres were equally preoccupied with dirt and disease. Well before the appearance of plague in Europe in 1347, towns and cities had a long tradition of sanitary legislation to deal with 'matter out of place'. The main aim was to address what was believed to be the cause of sickness, namely corrupt air, which came to be seen as containing within itself the 'seeds of disease'. Corrupt air or miasma was believed to be generated by stagnant pools or gases emitted from beneath the earth's surface through earthquakes, and then spread by wind to villages, towns and cities and thus infecting inhabitants with epidemic disease. Local factors specific to urban living conditions also produced corrupt air, such as industrial and domestic waste, exacerbated by people living in cramped, crowded conditions with inadequate systems of disposing of rubbish and human effluence. If governments found it more difficult to control earthquakes or strong winds, they could attempt to control the more local urban environment by passing laws to regulate the disposal of industrial and domestic waste prescribing for regular street sweeping, water supplies, and sewage disposal.

Recently a much clearer picture of the medieval city has emerged from studies of both northern and southern Europe, which have shown that both civic authorities and the public were involved in series of initiatives to keep the city cleaner than the image of the popular, modern imagination may suggest.[2] One of the main themes of medieval sanitary legislation was, as Rawcliffe shows in Chapter 1, the control of the butchery of animals since it was believed that this process led to the release of noxious vapours to contaminate the air and cause plague. In late medieval England, new purpose-built slaughterhouses were constructed on hygienic principles located outside the city centre to help prevent the production and increase of disease through corrupt air.[3]

It was this concern with corrupt vapours as causing and spreading disease which lay at the basis of the emergent plague legislation in the late medieval and early modern city. Beginning with street cleaning, digging large plague pits, and restrictions on the movement of people and goods, particularly cloth, which was seen as having the ability to hold within itself the corrupt vapours of disease, gradually a sophisticated system of quarantine and isolation developed, especially in the Italian peninsula. Massive lazaretti or isolation hospitals were established under the control of designated health boards, which over the centuries became permanent fixtures for the coordination of measures against potential causes and the threat of a range of epidemic diseases. Measures such as detailed sanitary surveys of housing and living conditions, as discussed by Henderson (Chapter 3, this volume), also emerged from the late sixteenth century onwards during periods of plague and typhus.[4]

Though plague was not the only disease to be linked to the city, it may be said to have functioned as a model of what Susan Craddock has called 'spatial pathologisation'.[5] Indeed plague measures, such as quarantine and sanitary cordons, have come to be seen as the model on which later measures against other epidemic diseases were based.[6] Many were founded on the central belief of the close relationship between corrupt air, smells, disease, and the urban fabric. These came to inform other environmental measures from the early eighteenth century onwards, such as the emergence of the new medical topographies across Europe, and the removal of cemeteries from the centre of the city, which in turn assumed a central role in broader social and political transformations.[7] By the nineteenth century, the connection of a range of pathologies with urban structures, textures, or ambiences became a question central to medical debates regarding the contagiousness of diseases.[8]

In the historiography of modern European and American urban pathologies, the cases of cholera and yellow fever are perhaps the most visible objects of concern: observations about the intimate relationship of both diseases to the urban environment was closely associated with arguments against their contagiousness. John Snow in his famous arguments on water-borne cholera (1849) had to fend off the criticisms of a barrage of physicians and medical officers, like William Farr, who were heavily invested in attributing cholera to the spatial order of London, to vapours and stenches associated with rising urban poverty.[9] Similarly, on the other side of the Atlantic Ocean, while 'smell detectives' roamed American cities in search of pathogens, debates about the aetiology of yellow fever drew heavily on the tropical conditions of Louisiana and New Orleans.[10] These argued that a local cause of the fevers was to be sought in the urban environment's exposure to the southern climatic conditions.[11] At the same time, on the American West Coast, dense living conditions and the impenetrable spaces of Chinatowns were seen as the principal source of smallpox outbreaks throughout the 1870s.[12] The entanglement of industrial urban living and the growing threat of tuberculosis became paradigmatic for connecting the urban environment with occupational diseases.[13] And finally syphilis, the great scourge of urban morality, became known as having reshaped the modernisation associated with urban space into a progressive condition of 'syphilisation'.[14]

By the close of the nineteenth century, the increased influence of medical geography had led epidemics to be regularly discussed both as global and urban disasters. Maps brought about a new visibility of the spaces of epidemics and in turn allowed a renewed scrutiny of the urban terrain as a place of infection.[15]

Looking beyond the well-trodden paths of the medical history of Europe and the USA, infectious disease control was catalytic to radical urban reforms in the Chinese treaty ports at the beginning of the twentieth century.[16] The spectre of cholera, and the civil unrest that habitually accompanied epidemics, led to the demolition of city walls, drying of moats, or the removal of cemeteries away from the centre of the city. Such reforms did not simply sanitise urban space, or make it easier to control and survey urban life; they also led to a destruction of the cosmological fabric of Chinese cities like Tianjin. Where these were originally structured and experienced on the basis of a complex cosmological order (including elements of Confucian ethics, geomancy, and cosmic-earthly analogy), they were now re-planned and retrofitted upon the image of 'hygienic modernity'.[17] Comparable developments can be observed in Latin America. The rising medical elites of Argentina, for example, took the prevalence of tuberculosis as the reason to develop an unprecedented programme of freeing the 'ailing city' from its scourge by planning and building parks and green land to integrate the healthy qualities of rural life.[18]

This biopolitical entanglement of the city with infectious diseases witnessed its apex in the context of colonial urban and medical planning, with the fifth and sixth cholera pandemics (1881–1896, 1899–1923) and the third plague pandemic (1894–1959). The city played a pivotal role in the pathologisation of native urban structures and modes of living, and in turn in 'spatial responses instigated to curtail the diffusion of disease', which led to complex shifts from enclavism, or the idea that elites could protect themselves from infection by isolating themselves from colonial subjects or the working classes, to public health measures.[19]

Such concerns have not diminished in contemporary times, though they have taken new forms, corresponding to current ideologies and scientific doctrines. Since the early 1990s, the rise of interest in emerging infectious diseases and the overall shift of focus from prevention to preparedness (as a Global Health doctrine that declares the outbreak of infectious diseases to be an inevitable event for which we can only be prepared), have led to the problematisation of the association of infectious diseases with forms of self-organised or spontaneous urbanisms, like slums or the 'wet markets' of East Asia.[20] At the same time, as recent crises like SARS and Ebola have brought quarantine and isolation back into practice, innovative approaches and designs of 'emergency urbanism' and 'preventative architecture' are on the rise.[21] These are seen not simply as a means of epidemic control, but explicitly as ways of 'defending the city'.[22] At the same time, the new focus on preparedness and its accompanying geographies of blame have rendered cities like Hong Kong into 'sentinels' of emerging infectious diseases, which it is feared may lead to the 'coming plague', as a mass contagion event leading to potential human extinction.[23] In popular culture this projected catastrophe has recently taken the form of films about pandemics framed in apocalyptic terms, where the image of abandoned cities, overtaken by 'nature', stand as evocative symbols of the end of human planetary domination, while at the same time producing a dystopian vision of the 'truly hygienic' city: one emptied of human life.

## The social life of plague

This volume seeks to underline the close connection between the city and plague. It examines how the disease was experienced and acted upon as arising from, unfolding in and challenging urban structures and urban life. This is not, of course, to deny the parallel association between rural areas and plague. To state the obvious, an epidemic had to arrive from somewhere and, when travelling across land and along trade and commercial routes, it passed through smaller settlements and the countryside, infecting local inhabitants and animals as it went. This is well exemplified by the arrival of plague in Florence in summer 1630, when it was carried by a chicken-dealer who returned home after selling chickens in infected parts of the Bolognese state (Henderson, Chapter 3, this volume). Indeed, Carlo Cipolla had already argued in 1981 that there were as high mortality rates from this epidemic in both rural and urban Tuscany.[24] More recently, Guido Alfani has placed Italian plague statistics within a European context and shown that during the seventeenth-century epidemics there were significantly higher levels of mortality in Italy compared with northern Europe. This phenomenon, he argues, is in part due to what he calls plague's 'exceptional territorial pervasiveness' in Italy, which felt its impact as much on many rural as urban areas, whereas in northern Europe plague had become a more exclusively urban phenomenon.[25] In other parts of the globe, and in Ottoman Anatolia and the Middle East, in particular, caravans spanning vast rural areas connected emerging cities in complex trading networks which may have enabled the spread of plague to both humans and animals.[26]

The other point which is related to the urban-rural context is how far it can be argued that plague was imported from or indeed originated in sylvatic reservoirs. More recently, ideas about plague's rural natural habitat date back to 1894 and to Russian research on the relation between plague and marmots in South Siberia.[27] If until recently momentous outbreaks of plague in urban centres have historiographically overshadowed the study of the development of endemic foci in the countryside and their long-term disease ecologies, the latter have started drawing sustained historical and anthropological attention. This has furthermore been enhanced by the advance of environmental historiography of disease landscapes.[28]

In examining the systematic linkage between urban space and plague, two things become immediately apparent. First, as seen above, the gradual evolution of plague measures in the late medieval and early modern European city led to the development of a panoply of prophylactic measures: from sanitary cordons and quarantine to public health boards and techniques of isolation. Then, at the same time, this urban focus fuelled policies of marginalisation and stigmatisation of economically and socially disadvantaged groups, to the point where the poor were seen as the cause of plague through their behaviour and consumption of food of poor quality leading to the corruption of their 'humours', which made up their body.[29]

While the third plague pandemic, which arose in China at the end of the nineteenth century, and which rapidly infected every inhabited continent, brought about a new ontology of plague based on its bacteriological identification, the disease continued to be treated as primarily an urban problem. Confirming recent critiques of the 'laboratory revolution' thesis, such as Michael Worboys' 'exclusive' sanitary reforms framework, Peter Baldwin's 'neo-quarantine' perspective and David Barnes' 'sanitary-bacteriological synthesis', not the laboratory, but notification, isolation, and disinfection assumed the primary role as measures against the disease.[30] Still, rather than being focused exclusively or primarily on human bodies, and hence marking a radical shift from previous counter-epidemic regimes, anti-plague operations continued to be equally applied to objects, infrastructures, and even the soil.[31]

This ever closer pathological association between plague and urban forms, structures and lifestyles was dependent on a 'materialisation of infection', which, as Graham Mooney has recently shown, conceived space as the locus of both public health risk and opportunity.[32] As plague science and policy developed within distinctly colonial medical frameworks, the defence of colonial cities against plague in Asia or Africa was understood as a defence of 'Europe', or more precisely of imperial metropoles.[33] At the same time, this global pandemic crisis also consolidated colony-to-colony connections, through the circulation of plague investigation and containment methods, plague researchers and plague-vanquishing military regiments between colonial cities and empires. These intricate networks of what Warwick Anderson has called 'biocolonial exchange' were further bolstered by international plague commissions and conferences, which helped consolidate and expand the association of plague and the urban environment as an object of both scientific knowledge and public health intervention.[34]

A fundamental theme that underlined the preoccupations and policies of local and international governments and organisations alike was the association between disease, poverty, and the urban environment. Centred on particular types of urban structures, such as narrow streets or windowless rooms, as well as features of urban life, such as close physical proximity, this process of pathologisation was reinvented (and reinvested) through distinct medical prisms across the centuries. Thus, in early modern Florence, as Henderson shows in Chapter 3, the city was likened to a body in which the living conditions of the poor were seen as fomenting the conditions to create plague. Contemporaries in seventeenth-century Tuscany were keen to problematise the close connection between disease and the conditions in which people lived.[35] In the words of Dr Antonio Pellicini, in his recommendations to the Health Board during the 1630–1631 epidemic of plague in Florence, such perspective necessitated a series of radical interventions:

> and remove those people shut up in houses, and especially the narrow evil shacks where there are a number of people living, not so much because of the many disorders which can take place, but because the enclosed air cannot be cleansed and is insalubrious.[36]

Yet, as Vanessa Harding points out in Chapter 2, studies of early modern London have shown that there was no consistent model in the correlation between the quality of housing and plague nor between poverty and plague across the series of outbreaks experienced by the city.[37]

The pathologisation of poor or working-class forms of habitation, especially as related to the urban terrain, remained the target of shifting understandings of plague. As Mary Sutphen has demonstrated in her study of plague in colonial Hong Kong and Calcutta, rendering the *where* rather than the *what* as the key question regarding plague allowed for a crucial synergy between different epidemiological schools at the turn of the nineteenth century, informing the persistence of 'contingent contagionism' after the bacteriological revolution.[38] In the case of Hong Kong, as discussed by Robert Peckham in Chapter 4, plague was associated with the city's Chinese 'coolie' neighbourhood of Taipingshan. James Lawson, the colony's chief medical officer, accordingly stated plague to be a 'poison' emanating from 'underneath houses', while Kitasato Shibasaburō, the first bacteriologist to claim to have isolated plague's pathogen, designated coolie houses as the ideal 'hunting grounds' for the bacillus.[39] In this manner, the bodies and objects of specific classes and races were configured as inhabiting urban space in ways that not only made them more vulnerable to plague but actually generated 'contagion'. A striking example of this is the association of the spread of plague with walking barefoot. Already in place in Hong Kong, but further developed in India, after the first outbreak of the disease in 1896, the idea was linked to the problematisation of the soil as a source of the disease.[40] No longer seen as a surface through which miasmatic gases from underlying putrefying matter escaped to infect humans, but as a bacteriological carrier of the pathogen, the soil remained the target of epidemiological suspicion as a 'breeding ground' of plague.

## Urban interventions

Over the centuries different modes of epidemic or pestilential control have configured the urban terrain. It may be perceived to be anachronistic to group these under the rubric of 'public health', but the phrase was certainly already used in seventeenth-century Italy, and more generally formed part of the much longer medieval and renaissance concept of the Common Good, which provided the ultimate justification of a state's raison d'être, to provide a safe and prosperous milieu for its subjects.[41]

Persistent strategies of combating plague have included sanitary legislation, quarantine (at home, in plague huts and on ships), isolation hospitals, sanitary cordons, cleansing, disinfecting and fumigating of private and public spaces, and even burning structures or areas believed to be harbouring the disease. Such interventions have taken particular forms derived from culturally specific understandings of disease and pollution. In her chapter on the urban environment in late medieval England, Carole Rawcliffe examines how ideas about the connection between urban practice, filth, and plague impacted on the urban landscape. As mentioned above, the key theme of Rawcliffe's chapter is the central preoccupation of urban authorities with the butchery of animals, and attempts were made to confine the

worst aspects of butchery to peripheral areas. The disposal of offal and other noxious waste taxed authorities to the limit, leading to the development of special
facilities for their removal, designed to protect the urban water supply and keep
the streets free of filth.

Over the centuries, underlying concepts linking plague and the city crossed
cultural borders to create types of intervention that by the end of the nineteenth
century would assume global proportions. Chinese dwellings became a key locus
of urban intervention against plague during the Third Pandemic. Plague made it
possible to penetrate the private space of Chinese houses and quarters and underlined its perceived connection to racialised perceptions of filth and stench. The
demolition of Chinese 'plague-haunted houses' in Hong Kong (Peckham, Chapter
4, this volume) and the officially sanctioned and meticulously planned burning of
'plagued houses' in Honolulu's Chinatown (Engelmann, Chapter 6, this volume)
were expressions of a racial anxiety, as described by Guenter Risse in the case of
San Francisco's Chinatown.[42] At the same time, such measures were grounded in
a contingent and open-ended aetiology, which merged bacteriological testing with
cultural stereotypes and miasmatic models of contagion.

The continuity of official measures across time was reflected in the meticulous
inspection of houses, recording their insanitary conditions and their classification as
'a cause of sickness' (Engelmann, Chapter 6, this volume) or as a source of corruption in early modern Florence (Henderson, Chapter 3, this volume). This provided
the rationale for drastic interventions in the urban sphere. More broadly, it led
public health in general, and plague in particular, to become catalysts for longer-
term urban reform. By the late nineteenth century, measures came to include
demolition, torching, retrofitting, segregation, and re-planning of the urban fabric.
The decision to adopt such drastic policies was often subject to public and expert
debate, as when the miasmatic and bacteriological ideas about plague aetiology
converged in the decision to demolish large areas of Taipingshan in Hong Kong.[43]
Furthermore, reference was often made to past outbreaks, so as to provide evidence for the best course of action. An example of this is when, in the first
years of the third plague pandemic, recourse to fire was linked explicitly to the
pervasive idea that the Great Fire of London in 1666 rid the city of plague.[44]
Indeed Harding (Chapter 2, this volume) suggests that one of the ways to better
understand the relationship between plague and the urban environment in early
modern London is to look at the structures and materials of housing. As plague
led to new perspectives on the life of the city, this also led to reconfigurations of
the urban environment. As Poleykett (Chapter 7, this volume) discusses in her
chapter on the plague-ridden cities of Rabat and Casablanca in the first decades of
the twentieth century, French colonial authorities adopted the Ville Moderne as
an anti-plague model in their Moroccan Protectorate. Plague outbreaks in these
cities challenged their status as showcases for a modern French urbanism. The
acclaimed achievements of sanitary measures, population-circulation control, and
aesthetisation became in turn examples of race, hygiene, and hierarchy in North
Africa, as plague reshaped knowledge about the urban space as much as about the

Moroccan body. This entanglement of plague, urban space, urban life, and the urban body was further articulated on the level of modes and tropes of visualising plague as a disease emanating from and threatening the urban milieu.

## Imagining and re-imagining plague

Visual representations of plague – and other epidemics – have long been under-stood as a visual afterlife of epidemic events, recording activities of containment or documenting suffering, destruction, and despair. Recent scholarship on visual history has shifted the perspective and emphasised the formative aspects of visual representations in the history of medicine.[45] Visual archives inform plague's historical narratives, pictures of plague apprehend, organise, and reveal outbreaks, and visual instruments were used to interrogate the divine sense or the biological shape of plague throughout history.[46] Crucially, pictures inform the relationship of plague to the urban environment. Just as the city works as a lens to look at the shape of plague, the epidemic and its continuous history can be used to map out urban space.[47] In the medieval and early modern periods, representations of plague took the form of the depiction of plague saints, such as St. Sebastian and St. Roch. Their role took two forms. They were either addressed as intercessors against a wrathful God to mitigate the impact of His punishment of mankind for their sins. Alternatively, saints received thanks for the cessation of plague, which led to the construction of churches, such as Santa Maria della Salute in Venice, to house the image of the Virgin. In both cases, the impact of plague on the urban environment tended to be shown either in the performance of a votive function or as a background for the performance of charitable works of a saintly figure, such as San Carlo Borromeo.[48] However, progressively, the city came to play an increasingly important role in depictions of the plague, whether it was in Nicholas Pousin's *The Plague of Ashdod* of 1630–1631 or Domenico Gargiulo's *Large del Marcatello during the Plague of 1656 in Naples* (1656–1660). Whereas each contained iconographic topoi which would have been familiar to contemporaries, such as the infant at the breast of the dead mother, both also placed their scenes of death and desolation firmly within an architectural urban context.[49] But it is the extraordinary series of prints by Louis Rouhier showing the measures taken in Rome during the plague of 1657 which really provides a detailed visual narrative through time and space of the development of the epidemic within its physical context. Each frame is linked by the constant movement of individuals and also groups of people as they move in processions from one part of the stricken city to another.[50] Appreciating the historical background of this iconographic tradition, the contributions to this volume move mostly beyond the established visual archive of plague to emphasise new conventions and the introduction of a renewed aesthetic of plague through photography in the third plague pandemic.

Photography placed the epidemic's visual representation between the poles of scientific reasoning and popular imagination, merging artistic and historical imaginations in the perception of objective, mechanical reproductions. Thus, new visual repositories were integrated into the image of plague. They merged, for example, the symbolic position of the ruin as a representation of late Qing China as a decaying empire with the Chinese dwelling to reveal the 'plague-ruin' as a cornerstone of the photographic sanitary regime in Hong Kong. In his Chapter 4, Robert Peckham describes how plague photography thus merged colonial power with the sanitary policy applied to the plague house in the British Empire. The visualisation of Chinatown is equally of interest to Engelmann (Chapter 6, this volume), who focuses on photographic renderings of plagued houses in 1899–1900 Hawaii. Drawing on the association between medical photographic practices and the rationality of disease geography and clinical portraiture, he exposes the unusual and often overlooked application of photography to the visualisation of plague spaces in the urban setting of Honolulu's Chinatown. The extensive albums of photographed plague houses in Honolulu foregrounded ecological disease models, and enhanced a complex understanding of plague between bacterial agents, human hosts, and the urban terrain, to provide visual evidence that justified the destruction of dwellings in the name of public health.

The visual representation of the third plague pandemic thus stands in sharp contrast to the visual archives of plague's long history. Unlike medieval and renaissance painting, plague photography was rarely deployed to visualise sick bodies of plague victims; it became instead a standardised medium to capture large numbers of dwellings connected to incidences of plague. An emphasis on the space through which plague is understood is also reflected in the use of disease mapping. The cartography of the urban milieu of disease, as, for example, in John Snow's famous cholera map, does build on the representation of preventive measures against plague, as in the maps of sanitary cordons dating from the last throws of the second plague pandemic in southern Europe.[51] This was much further developed in the colonial urban context and forms an important part of Evans' contribution to this volume (Chapter 5) on a particular plague map of a small fishing village in Bombay, published in 1897. Whereas infection and human to human transmission became the predominant frame of colonial authority's perception of the Indian urban space, the map took up a crucial position as synthesiser of grouped plague cases. Plotting plague onto the colonial fantasy of space and landscape reveals first and foremost the failure of arriving at a clear picture of the epidemic. Instead of certitude about plague, the map emphasised the inherent fragility of the colonial sanitary regime in British India. Plague underlined the structural instability of colonial power, not only in India but also, as Poleykett demonstrates (Chapter 7, this volume), in Rabat and Casablanca. Plague's persistence, despite the showcasing of the Moroccan cities as examples of French Modernism, constituted both a scandal and a constant planning heuristic, which reshaped knowledge about the spaces and dispositions of the Moroccan body in the city.

Studies of visual representations, urban planning, sanitary legislation, and the discernment of soil, stench, and dirt have been brought together in this volume around a concern about plague's invisibility. The regulations of stench in late medieval England (Rawcliffe, Chapter 1, this volume) and the problematisation of dirt in early modern Florence (Henderson, Chapter 3, this volume) underline a longstanding concern with the 'invisible enemy': reflected through the employment over the centuries of orders, tables, registers, drawings, maps, petri-dishes, caricatures, and photographs.[52] Often seen as a 'concealed' disease, through the pathogen's supposed ability to hide or lay latent for long periods of time, and some members of society's alleged propensity to hide plague cases from authorities, from the middle ages to the colonial period, plague became subject to what Lynteris has described elsewhere as both a demonstrative and forensic photographic faculty.[53] While demonstrative photography treated the urban terrain as a scene where the breeding grounds, transmission pathways, and origin of plague could be visualised, photography's forensic faculty visualised different urban forms as elements of the invisibility of plague, making the disease everywhere implied but nowhere to be seen. Photographic productions, such as the one examined by Engelmann, or Williamson's San Francisco Chinatown photographic album for the local Board of Health, were meant to construct albums of suspect-as-pathogenic areas, creating series of sites and sights implicated in incidents of plague.[54] On the one hand, this total archive was supposed to allow future scientists to decipher the cause of a given outbreak (with the help of new, yet unforeseen and unavailable clues), and, on the other hand, to generate an image of Honolulu or San Francisco's Chinatowns as urban ecologies of plague.[55]

## Conclusion

The contributions to this volume reveal urban space as a complex social and epistemological terrain of bubonic plague. The understanding of different historical articulations of plague as an urban phenomenon requires the adoption of analytical perspectives that go beyond well-trodden continuity–discontinuity dichotomies in the history of public health. Plague was associated in different times and contexts with filth, stench, impoverished lifestyles, wooden, and brick structures, infected soils, as well as with class and race stereotypes. It was combatted through fire, quarantine, isolation, disinfection, and urban re-planning. This urban history of plague is examined here in terms of its rich social, political, scientific, medical, and visual imprint. The decisive impact of the city on the history of plague is examined in this volume through perspectives that incorporate not only different historical periods, but also approaches from visual studies, history of public health, urban studies, society and medicine, philosophy of science, postcolonial studies, and anthropology. The assembled perspectives thus emphasise that the medical history of plague is not just the history of its medicine.

## Acknowledgements

Research leading to this Introduction was funded by a European Research Council Starting Grant (under the European Union's Seventh Framework Programme/ ERC grant agreement no 336564) for the project Visual Representations of the

Third Plague Pandemic. We would like to thank the participants of the conference 'Plague and the City: Disease, Epidemic Control and the Urban Environment' (CRASSH, University of Cambridge, UK) for their generous feedback on the questions regarding the topic of this volume.

## Notes

1   Bradley (ed.), *Rome, Pollution and Propriety*; Douglas, *Purity and Danger*.
2   Rawcliffe, *Urban Bodies*; Geltner, 'Healthscaping a Medieval City'.
3   Rawcliffe, *Urban Bodies*; and on Tuscany: Cipolla, *Miasmas and Disease*; Zagli *et al.*, *Maladetti beccari*.
4   Cipolla, *Miasmas and Disease*; Carmichael, *Plague and the Poor*; Cipolla, *Public Health*.
5   Craddock, *City of Plagues*.
6   Bashford, *Imperial Hygiene*.
7   Riley, *The Eighteenth-Century Campaign*; Dobson, *Contours of Death*; Elden, 'Plague, Panopticon, Police'; Foucault, *Discipline and Punish*.
8   Barnes, *The Great Stink of Paris*.
9   Eyler, *Victorian Social Medicine*; Gilbert, *Mapping the Victorian Social Body*.
10  Kielche, *Smell Detectives*.
11  Coleman, *Yellow Fever in the North*; Humphreys, *Yellow Fever and the South*.
12  Shah, *Contagious Divides*.
13  Dubos, Dubos, *The White Plague*; Condrau and Worboys, *Tuberculosis Then and Now*.
14  Quetel, *History of Syphilis*, 112–114.
15  Hirsch, *Handbook*; Koch, *Disease Maps*; Shah, *Contagious Divides*.
16  Rosenberg, *The Cholera Years*; Whooley, *Knowledge in the Time of Cholera*.
17  Rogaski, *Hygienic Modernity*.
18  Armus, *The Ailing City*; Engelmann, 'Fumigating the Model Hygienic City'.
19  Wald, '"Global Health"', 217; On enclavism and the need to move beyond teleological historiographies of its shift to public health see: Peckham and Pomfert, 'Introduction'.
20  Lakoff, *Unprepared*; Lynteris, 'The Prophetic Faculty of Epidemic Photography'.
21  Sample, 'Emergency Urbanism and Preventative Architecture'.
22  *Ibid.*, 247.
23  Keck, 'From Purgatory to Sentinel: 'Forms/Events' in the Field of Zoonoses'.
24  Cipolla, Fighting the Plague, 100–103.
25  Alfani, *Calamities*; *ibid.*, 'Wealth Inequalities'; Alfani and Cohn, 'Nonontola'.
26  Varlik, Plague and Empire in the Early Modern Mediterranean World.
27  Lynteris, *Ethnographic Plague*.
28  Ziegler, 'Landscapes of Disease'.
29  Henderson, Chapter 3, this volume; more broadly: Wear, *Knowledge and Practice in English Medicine*; Pullan, 'Plague and Perceptions of the Poor in Early Modern Italy'.
30  Baldwin, *Contagion and the State in Europe*; Barnes, *The Great Stink of Paris*; Worboys, *Spreading Germs*.
31  Peckham, 'Hong Kong Junk'; Lynteris, 'A Suitable Soil'.
32  Mooney, *Intrusive Interventions*, 15.
33  See in particular, Proust, *La défense de l'Europe*.
34  Anderson, 'The Possession of Kuru'.
35  Cipolla, *Miasmas and Disease*.
36  Pellicini, *Discorso sopra di mali contagiosi pestilenziali*.
37  Champion, *London's Dreaded Visitation*; Cummins, Kelly, and Grada, 'Living Standards and Plague in London, 1560–1665'.
38  Kidambi, '"An Infection of Locality"', 251; Sutphen, 'Not What, but Where'.
39  Lowson, Handwritten report; Kitasato, 'The Bacillus of Bubonic Plague'.
40  Lynteris, 'A Suitable Soil'.

41 Archivio di Stato di Firenze, Sanità, Negozi 154, f. 205r: 15.1.1631, in a letter written by Father Donato Bisogni to the Florentine Health Board about his time as director of the Lazaretto of San Miniato: 'I have dedicated every hour to the service of the public health [pubblica salute]'. On ideas of the Common Good as applied to poor relief see, Henderson, *Piety and Charity*, 16–20, 344–359. Rosen, Martí-Ibáñez, *A History of Public Health*; Cipolla, *Miasmas and Disease*.

42 Risse, *Plague, Fear, and Politics.*

43 Sutphen, 'Not What but Where'.

44 Lynteris, 'A Suitable Soil'.

45 Daston and Galison, 'The Image of Objectivity'; Mitchell, *What Do Pictures Want?*; Tucker, *Nature Exposed*; Wilder, *Photography and Science*; Serlin (ed.), *Imagining Illness*; Engelmann, 'Photographing AIDS'.

46 Poleykett, Evans, Engelmann, 'Fragments of Plague'.

47 Shah, *Contagious Divides.*

48 For a comprehensive overview, see, Boeckl, *Images of Plague and Pestilence*; Fox and Karp, 'Images of Plague'; Marshall, 'Manipulating the Sacred'; Power, 'Media Dependency'.

49 Barker, 'Poussin, Plague and Early Modern Medicine', 669; Clifton, 'Art and Plague at Naples', 113.

50 San Juan, *Rome: A City out of Print*, Chapter 7.

51 McLeod, 'Our Sense of Snow'; Cliff, Smallman-Raynor, and Stevens, 'Controlling the Geographical Spread of Infectious Disease'; Jarcho, 'Some Early Italian Epidemiological Maps'.

52 Cipolla, *Public Health*, 39.

53 Lynteris, 'The Prophetic Faculty of Epidemic Photography'.

54 Williamson Album at San Francisco Public Library (uncatalogued, no call number); see Risse, *Plague, Fear, and Politics* for a selection of captions.

55 For a discussion of archives of the future in the sciences, see Daston, 'The Sciences of the Archive'. On the notion of the total archive see, Jardine and Kelly (eds.), 'The Total Archive'.

# References

## Primary sources

Archivio di Stato di Firenze, Sanità, Negozi, 154.

Lowson, James A., Handwritten report, 16 May 1894, enclosed in Robinson to Ripon, 17 May 1894. Original Correspondence, 1841–1951; Series 129/263, CO 10928 (Hong Kong: Colonial Office).

Pellicini, Antonio, *Discorso sopra di mali contagiosi pestilenziali* (Florence: Zanobi Pignoni, 1630), 14.

Williamson Album at San Francisco Public Library (uncatalogued, no call number).

## Secondary sources

Alfani, Guido, *Calamities and the Economy in Renaissance Italy: The Grand Tour of the Horsemen of the Apocalypse* (Basingstoke: Palgrave Macmillan, 2013).

Alfani, Guido, 'Wealth Inequalities and Population Dynamics in Early Modern Northern Italy', *Journal of Interdisciplinary History*, 40 (2010), 513–549.

Alfani, Guido and Samuel Cohn, 'Nonontola, 1630: Anatomia di una pestilenzia meccanismi del contagio', *Popolazione e Storia*, 2 (2007), 99–138.

Anderson, Warwick, 'The Possession of Kuru: Medical Science and Biocolonial Exchange', *Comparative Studies in Society and History*, 42, 4 (2000), 713–744.

Armus, Diego, *The Ailing City: Health, Tuberculosis, and Culture in Buenos Aires, 1870–1950* (Durham, NC: Duke University Press, 2011).

Baldwin, Peter, *Contagion and the State in Europe, 1830–1930* (Cambridge, UK: Cambridge University Press, 1999).

Barker, Sheila, 'Poussin, Plague and Early Modern Medicine', *The Art Bulletin*, 86, 4 (2004), 659–689.

Barnes, David S., *The Great Stink of Paris and the Nineteenth-Century Struggle Against Filth and Germs* (Baltimore: Johns Hopkins University Press, 2006).

Bashford, Alison, *Imperial Hygiene: A Critical History of Colonialism, Nationalism and Public Health* (Basingstoke: Palgrave Macmillan, 2004).

Boeckl, Christine M., *Images of Plague and Pestilence: Iconology and Iconology* (Missouri: Truman State University Press, 2000).

Bradley, Mark (ed.), *Rome, Pollution and Propriety: Dirt, Disease and Hygiene in the Eternal City from Antiquity to Modernity* (Cambridge, UK: Cambridge University Press, 2012).

Carmichael, Ann G., *Plague and the Poor in Renaissance Florence* (Cambridge, UK: Cambridge University Press, 1986).

Champion, Justin A.I., *London's Dreaded Visitation: The Social Geography of the Great Plague in 1665* (London: Centre of Metropolitan History, 1995).

Cipolla, Carlo M., *Fighting the Plague in Seventeenth-Century Italy* (Madison: University of Wisconsin Press, 1981).

Cipolla, Carlo M., *Miasmas and Disease: Public Health and the Environment in the Pre-Industrial Age* (New Haven and London: Yale University Press, 1992).

Cipolla, Carlo M., *Public Health and the Medical Profession in the Renaissance* (Cambridge, UK: Cambridge University Press, 1976).

Cliff, Andrew D., Matthew R. Smallman-Raynor, and Peta M. Stevens, 'Controlling the Geographical Spread of Infectious Disease: Plague in Italy, 1347–1851', *Acta Medico-Historica Adriatica*, 7, 1 (2009), 197–236.

Clifton, James, 'Art and Plague at Naples', in: Gauvin Alexander Bailey, Pamela M. Jones, F. Mormando, and Thomas W. Worcester (eds.), *Hope and Healing: Painting in Italy in a Time of Plague, 1500–1800* (Chicago: Chicago University Press, 2005), 97–117.

Coleman, William, *Yellow Fever in the North: The Methods of Early Epidemiology* (Madison: University of Wisconsin Press, 1987).

Condrau, Flurin and Michael Worboys, *Tuberculosis Then and Now: Perspectives on the History of an Infectious Disease* (Kingston: McGill Queen's University Press, 2010).

Craddock, Susan, *City of Plagues: Disease, Poverty, and Deviance in San Francisco* (Minneapolis: University of Minnesota Press, 2004).

Cummins, Neil, Morgan Kelly, and Cormac Ó Grada, 'Living Standards and Plague in London, 1560–1665', *Economic History Review*, 69, 1 (2015), 3–34.

Daston, Lorraine, 'The Sciences of the Archive', *Osiris*, 27, 1 (2012), 156–187.

Daston, Lorraine and Peter Galison, 'The Image of Objectivity', *Representations, Special Issue: Seeing Science*, 40, (1992), 81–128.

Dobson, Mary, J., *Contours of Death and Disease in Early Modern England* (Cambridge, UK: Cambridge University Press, 1997).

Douglas, Mary, *Purity and Danger: An Analysis of Concepts of Pollution and Taboo* (London: Routledge, 2003 [1966]).

Dubos, René Jules, and Jean Dubos, *The White Plague: Tuberculosis, Man, and Society* (New Brunswick: Rutgers University Press, 1952).

Elden, Stuart, 'Plague, Panopticon, Police', *Surveillance & Society*, 1, 3 (2002), 240–253.

Engelmann, Lukas, 'Fumigating the Model Hygienic City: Bubonic Plague and the Sulfurozador in Early-Twentieth Century Buenos Aires', *Medical History*, 62, 3 (2018), n.p.

Engelmann, Lukas, 'Photographing AIDS: Capturing AIDS in Pictures of People with AIDS', *Bulletin of the History of Medicine*, 90, 2 (2016), 250–278.

Eyler, John M., *Victorian Social Medicine: The Ideas and Methods of William Farr* (Cambridge, UK: Cambridge University Press, 1979).

Foucault, Michel, *Discipline and Punish: The Birth of the Prison* (London: Vintage Books, 1977)

Fox, Daniel M. and D. R. Karp, 'Images of Plague: Infectious Disease in the Visual Arts', in: Elizabeth Fee and Daniel M. Fox (eds.), *AIDS: The Burdens of History* (Berkeley: University of California Press, 1988), 172–189.

Geltner, Guy, 'Healthscaping a Medieval City: Lucca's *Curia viarum* and the Future of Public Health', *Urban History*, 40 (2015), 395–415.

Gilbert, Pamela K., *Mapping the Victorian Social Body* (New York: State University of New York Press, 2004).

Henderson, John, *Piety and Charity in Late Medieval Florence* (Oxford: Oxford University Press, 1994).

Hirsch, August, *Handbook of Geographical and Historical Pathology* (London: New Sydenham Society, 1883).

Humphreys, Margaret, *Yellow Fever and the South* (Baltimore: Johns Hopkins University Press, 1999).

Jarcho, Saul, 'Some Early Italian Epidemiological Maps', *Imago Mundi*, 35, 1 (1983), 9–19.

Jardine, Boris and Christopher Kelly (eds.), 'The Total Archive', *Limn* 6 (March 2016): http://limn.it/issue/06/.

Juan, Rose Maria San, *Rome: A City Out of Print* (Minneapolis: University of Minnesota Press, 2001).

Keck, Frédéric, 'From Purgatory to Sentinel: "Forms/Events" in the Field of Zoonoses', *Cambridge Anthropology*, 32, 1 (2014), 47–61.

Kidambi, Prashant, '"An Infection of Locality": Plague, Pythogenesis and the Poor in Bombay, 1896–1905', *Urban History*, 31, 2 (2004), 249–267.

Kielche, Melanie, A., *Smell Detectives: An Olfactory History of Nineteenth-Century Urban America* (Washington, DC: University of Washington Press, 2017).

Kitasato, S., 'The Bacillus of Bubonic Plague', *Lancet*, 144, 3704 (1894), 428–430.

Koch, Tom, *Disease Maps: Epidemics on the Ground* (Chicago: University of Chicago Press, 2011).

Kosoy, Michael and Roman Kosoy, 'Complexity and Biosemiotics in Evolutionary Ecology of Zoonotic Infectious Agents', *Evolutionary Applications*, 11 (2018), 394–403.

Lakoff, Andrew, *Unprepared: Global Health in a Time of Emergency* (Berkeley: The University of California Press, 2017).

Lynteris, Christos, 'The Prophetic Faculty of Epidemic Photography: Chinese Wet Markets and the Imagination of the Next Pandemic', *Visual Anthropology*, 29, 2 (2016), 118–132.

Lynteris, Christos, 'A Suitable Soil: Plague's Breeding Grounds at the Dawn of the Third Pandemic', *Medical History*, 61, 3 (2017), 343–357.

Lynteris, Christos, *Ethnographic Plague: Configuring Disease on the Chinese-Russian Frontier* (London: Palgrave Macmillan, 2016).

Marshall, Louise, 'Manipulating the Sacred: Image and Plague in Renaissance Italy', *Renaissance Quarterly*, 47, 3 (1994), 485–532.

McLeod, Kari S., 'Our Sense of Snow: The Myth of John Snow in Medical Geography', *Social Science & Medicine*, 50, 7 (2000), 923–935.

Mitchell, W. J. T., *What Do Pictures Want? The Lives and Loves of Images* (Chicago: University of Chicago Press, 2005).

Mooney, Graham, *Intrusive Interventions. Public Health, Domestic Space, and Infectious Disease Surveillance in England, 1840–1914* (Rochester, NY: University of Rochester Press, 2015).

Peckham, Robert, 'Hong Kong Junk: Plague and the Economy of Chinese Things', *Bulletin of the History of Medicine*, 90 (2016): 32–60.

Peckham, Robert and David M. Pomfert, 'Introduction: Medicine, Hygiene and the Re-Ordering of Empire', in: Robert Peckham and David M. Pomfert, (eds.), *Imperial Contagions: Medicine, Hygiene, and Cultures of Planning in Asia* (Hong Kong: Hong Kong University Press, 2013), 1–16.

Poleykett, Branwyn, Nicholas H. A. Evans, and Lukas Engelmann, 'Fragments of Plague', *Limn* 6 (March 2016): http://limn.it/fragments-of-plague/.

Power, J. G., 'Media Dependency, Bubonic Plague, and the Social Construction of the Chinese Other', *Journal of Communication Inquiry*, 19, 1 (1995), 89–110.

Pullan, Brian, 'Plague and Perceptions of the Poor in Early Modern Italy', in: T. Ranger and P. Slack, (eds.), *Epidemics and Ideas* (Cambridge, UK: Cambridge University Press, 1992), 101–123.

Proust, A., *La défense de l'Europe contre la peste et la conférence de Venise de 1897* (Paris: Masson et Cie, 1897).

Quétel, Claude, *History of Syphilis* (Cambridge, UK: Polity Press, 1990).

Rawcliffe, Carole, *Urban Bodies. Communal Health in Late Medieval English Towns and Cities* (Woodbridge: The Boydell Press, 2013).

Riley, James C., *The Eighteenth-Century Campaign to Avoid Disease* (Basingstoke: Macmillan, 1987).

Risse, Guenter B., *Plague, Fear, and Politics in San Francisco's Chinatown* (Baltimore and London: Johns Hopkins University Press, 2012).

Rogaski, Ruth, *Hygienic Modernity; Meanings of Health and Disease in Treaty-Port China* (Berkeley: University of California Press, 2004).

Rosen, George and Félix Martí-Ibáñez, *A History of Public Health* (New York: MD Publications, 1958).

Rosenberg, Charles E., *The Cholera Years. The United States in 1832, 1849, and 1866* (Chicago: University of Chicago Press, 1962).

Sample, H., 'Emergency Urbanism and Preventative Architecture', in: G. Borasi and M. Zardini (eds.), *Imperfect Health: The Medicalization of Architecture* (Kosler: Canadian Centre for Architecture/Lars Muller Publishers, 2012), 231–249.

Serlin, David Harley (ed.), *Imagining Illness. Public Health and Visual Culture* (Minneapolis: University of Minnesota Press, 2010).

Shah, Nayan, *Contagious Divides: Epidemics and Race in San Francisco's Chinatown* (Berkeley: University of California Press, 2001).

Sutphen, Mary P., 'Not What, but Where: Bubonic Plague and the Reception of Germ Theories in Hong Kong and Calcutta', *Journal of History of Medicine and Allied Sciences*, 52, 1 (1997), 81–113.

Tucker, Jennifer, *Nature Exposed: Photography as Eyewitness in Victorian Science* (Baltimore: Johns Hopkins University Press, 2005).

Varlik, Nukhet, *Plague and Empire in the Early Modern Mediterranean World* (Cambridge, UK: Cambridge University Press, 2015).

Wald, Priscilla, '"Global Health" and the Persistence of History', in: Robert Peckham and David M. Pomfret (eds.), *Imperial Contagions: Medicine, Hygiene, and Cultures of Planning in Asia* (Hong Kong: Hong Kong University Press, 2013), 215–226.

Wear, Andrew, *Knowledge and Practice in English Medicine, 1550–1680* (Cambridge, UK: Cambridge University Press, 2000).

Whooley, Owen, *Knowledge in the Time of Cholera: The Struggle over American Medicine in the Nineteenth Century* (Chicago: University of Chicago Press, 2013).

Wilder, Kelley E., *Photography and Science* (London: Reaktion, 2009).

Worboys, Michael, *Spreading Germs: Disease Theories and Medical Practice in Britain, 1865–1900* (Cambridge, UK: Cambridge University Press, 2000).

Zagli, Andrea, Francesco Mineccia, and Andrea Giuntini, *Maladetti beccari: storia dei macellari fiorentini dal Cinquescento al Duemila* (Florence: Polistampa, 2000).

Ziegler, Michelle, 'Landscapes of Disease', *Landscapes*, 17, 2 (2016), 99–107.

# 1

# 'GREAT STENCHES, HORRIBLE SIGHTS, AND DEADLY ABOMINATIONS'

## Butchery and the battle against plague in late medieval English towns

*Carole Rawcliffe*

In early January 1350 as the people of Norwich were counting the cost of their first devastating experience of bubonic plague, the bailiffs' court, then the most important judicial body in the city, resumed its hearings. Not surprisingly, given the recent level of disruption and scale of mortality, few individuals then faced prosecution, but one case, in particular, attracts attention, not least for the severity of the sentence. It concerns a local butcher named William Brok, who was found guilty of selling 'meat of oxen and sheep measly, bad and putrid through age' (*succematas corruptas et pro vetustate putridas*). The offending wares were to be burnt, while Brok himself was to be imprisoned at the court's pleasure, but only after spending an unspecified time in the public pillory.[1] We do not know if, as was already the case in London, the rotting meat was actually burnt beneath him as he endured this very public humiliation, but at a slightly later date corrupt foodstuffs were customarily destroyed on a bonfire in the middle of Norwich market, right next to the pillory.[2]

It was certainly appropriate that one whose merchandise had polluted the environment and endangered the lives of his fellow citizens should be obliged to inhale the noxious fumes of contaminated meat. For, in the context of a community recently ravaged by pestilence, Brok's conduct must have seemed little short of homicidal, as other contemporary urban records confirm. One of the very first measures instituted by the rulers of Venice when plague struck in 1348 was to order the incineration of infected pork, 'which creates a great stench and attendant putrefaction that corrupts the air'.[3] Ordinances passed by the mayor and aldermen of London in the aftermath of the second great national epidemic of 1361–1362 specifically warned victuallers against retaining foodstuffs until they became 'corrupt and stinking', upon pain of the draconian punishment just described.[4]

This chapter will explore the ways in which a steadily growing body of regulations for the control of butchers and butchery in late medieval English

towns can illuminate and develop our knowledge of urban responses to epidemic disease. Having established the extent to which the populace at large
acquired a working knowledge of relatively sophisticated and complex theories
about human physiology, it will concentrate upon the impact of these ideas upon
the built environment. We can detect a close relationship between the fear of
plague and the creation of purpose-built slaughterhouses and meat markets, the
introduction of designated refuse-disposal systems and the practical steps taken
to safeguard water supplies from contamination by blood and offal. Systematic
attempts were also made to oversee the quality of the urban meat supply through
the more stringent inspection of markets and introduction of byelaws designed
to eliminate insanitary practices.

A few scholars have already drawn specific attention to some of these initiatives: one of the three pioneering articles on public health in fourteenth-century
London published in the 1930s by Ernest Sabine focused upon the city's butchers. Although he did not attempt to place the measures that he described within
the wider context of contemporary medical beliefs, Sabine was convinced that
there must have been 'some correlation' between them and 'the ravages of the
Black Death'. He also felt it important to document the efforts made by the civic
authorities to curb pollution and protect the community as a whole.[5] Both Philip
Jones and David Carr have reiterated this message, the former in an official history
of the Butchers' Company of London in which he approvingly documents various
early campaigns 'to improve sanitary conditions'. He does not, however, consider
*why* 'the dangers of contamination and contagion' came to be so closely associated
with unregulated butchery, or explore any possible connections between fear of
infection and the imposition of tighter controls.[6] Carr's brief survey of the ways
in which late medieval English towns dealt with their butchers resorts to similar
generalisations. While maintaining that magistrates were primarily motived by a
'simple desire to have a more pleasant, more "respectable" urban environment',
he nevertheless concedes – without further elaboration – that a contemporary
'myth' attributing the spread of disease to airborne miasmas may also have gained
'broad acceptance'.[7]

Despite the appearance of a rapidly growing corpus of publications that
explores this 'myth' and its impact on late medieval strategies for the preservation of communal health,[8] the assumption that men and women (and especially
*English* men and women) remained supine in the face of pestilence still persists in
some academic circles. As recently as 2012, Ole Benedictow argued that it was
not until the sixteenth century that people ceased to accept epidemics 'fatalisti-
cally as a divine punishment for human sin' and began to regard them as a 'natural
phenomenon . . . that could be prevented, limited or halted by human counter-
measures'.[9] It would be foolish to deny that plague was, ultimately, regarded
as an act of divine retribution (which might, significantly, be assuaged through
charitable works, such as the provision of refuse-disposal systems), but we need
also to recognise that more immediate and potentially more manageable agents
seemed also to be involved.[10]

## Butchery and the transmission of plague

Chief among these agents was corrupt air, which had long been blamed for the spread of epidemics and was frequently associated with the stench arising from butchers' waste. Indeed, the vernacular plague tracts or *concilia* which circulated in increasing numbers during the late fourteenth and fifteenth century warned specifically against the threat posed by 'stynken caryn cast in the water nye to the cytees or townes, as the boles [entrails] of bestes'.[11] The reader was consequently urged 'to eschew halle euyl aers [all evil air], as to say in stabulys, ffyldys & strettys & namely the heer [air] of bestys that soddenly dye & be stynkyng'.[12] Advice manuals of this kind drew heavily on the *Canon* of Avicenna, which had formed the bedrock of the European medical syllabus since the thirteenth century. An influential passage in book four describes the toxic effect of miasmatic exhalations upon the human body:

> Vapours and fumes rise [into the air] and spread in it, and putrefy it with their debilitating warmth. And when air of this kind reaches the heart, it corrupts the complexion of the spirit that dwells within it; and, surrounding the heart, it then putrefies it with humidity. And there arises an unnatural heat; and it spreads throughout the body, as a result of which pestilential fever will occur, and will spread to a multitude of men who likewise have vulnerable dispositions.[13]

Shorn of their theoretical underpinnings, these ideas began to percolate downwards through society at a comparatively early date, their transmission (often through the medium of statutes, royal ordinances, civic proclamations, and local byelaws) being hastened by repeated outbreaks of plague from the 1360s onwards.[14] It is hardly surprising that the University authorities in Cambridge, who knew their Avicenna, should insist in the aftermath of the fourth national pestilence of 1374–1375 that all 'putrid flesh' and other noxious waste had to be removed from the butchers' shops every morning and evening. Even so, their response was far from unusual.[15]

Notwithstanding the fact that London's three major meat markets and slaughterhouses had already been consigned to peripheral areas, including St. Nicholas Shambles at Newgate (see the map in Figure 1.1), we can readily appreciate why Edward III prohibited the butchering of animals anywhere near the city during the second and third great national epidemics of 1361–1362 and 1368–1369. His attempts permanently to remove such activities to Knightsbridge (in the west) and Stratford (in the north-east) nonetheless had unwelcome consequences and encountered widespread resistance. Whereas some butchers raised their prices to allow for the cost of transport, thereby occasioning disturbances in the city, others took the easy option of dumping their offal immediately outside the walls in the watercourses, fields, and ditches of Holborn.[16] The ensuing outcry by a group of influential courtiers and other prominent local residents reflects a timeless desire on the part of affluent householders to preserve the value of their property. But a real

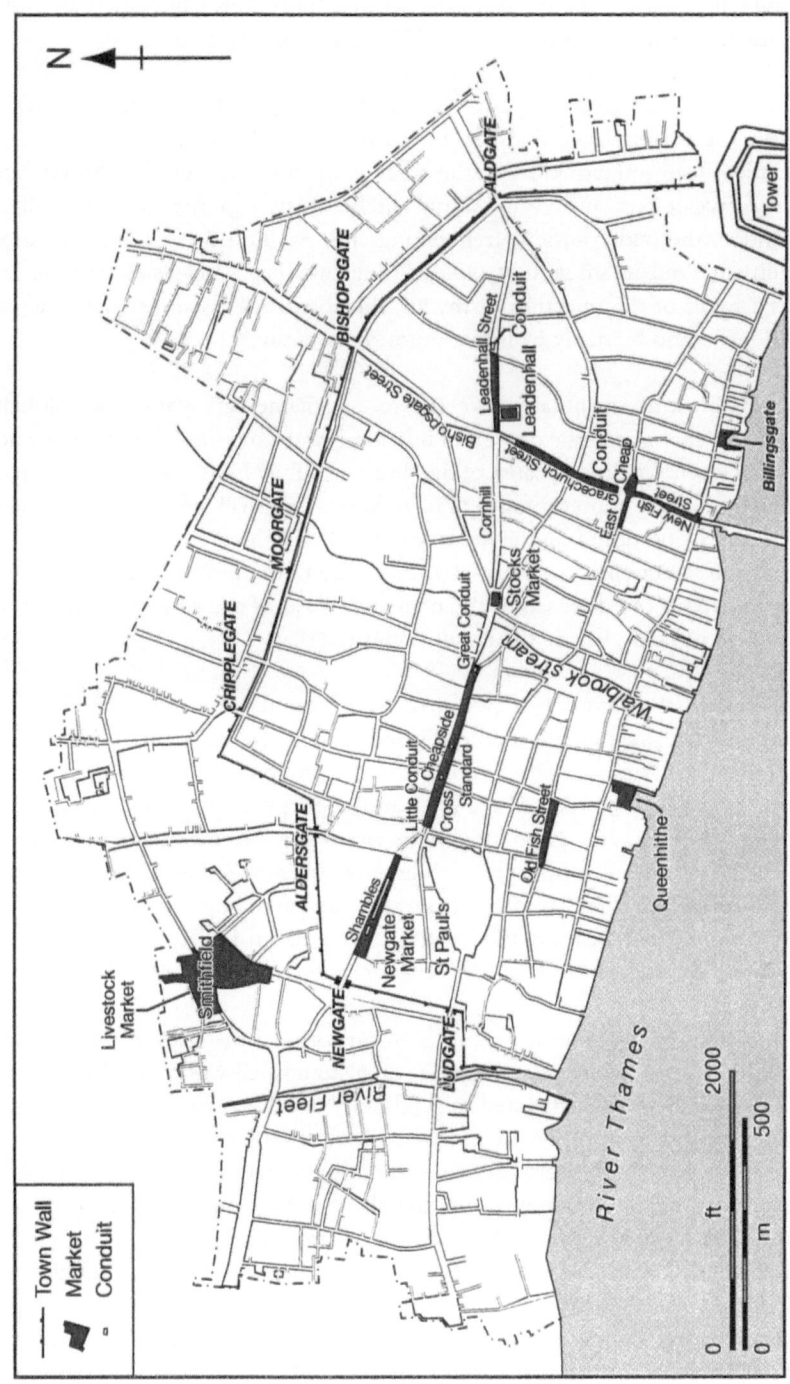

**FIGURE 1.1** Map of the markets and butcheries of late medieval London

Drawn by Cath D'Alton, to whom we are grateful for permission to reproduce it here

fear of infection is also apparent from the petition for redress which they submitted to parliament during the plague year of 1379, complaining that:

> because of the great and horrible stenches and deadly abominations which arise there from day to day from the corrupt blood [*sank corrupt*] and entrails of cattle, sheep and pigs killed in the butchery next to the church of St. Nicholas in Newgate and thrown in various ditches in two gardens near to Holborn Bridge, the said courtiers, frequenting and dwelling there, contract various ailments, and are grievously exposed to disease [*trop grevousement mys a disease*] as a result of the infection of the air, the abominations and stenches above-said, and also by many evils that notoriously ensue.[17]

Protests of this kind eventually gave rise to a parliamentary statute of 1388 that comprehensively forbade the deposit of butchers' waste and similar refuse in or near *any* English towns or cities because of the threat to public health posed by miasmatic air.[18] The translation of precept into practice was, as we shall see, harder to achieve, but there can be no doubting the sanitary imperative behind this legislation.[19]

Even more eloquent, a petition of 1372 to the Crown from York's Franciscan community about the disposal of 'the offal and blood of great beasts' in the River Ouse and on its banks below their walls, reported that:

> the air in their church is poisoned by the stench there generated as well around the altars where the Lord's body is daily ministered as in other their houses, and flies and other vermin are thereby bred and enter their church and houses, so that as well the lords and noble persons of the country flocking to the city as the good men of the city who used to come to their church to hear mass and to pray are withdrawing themselves because of the stench and *the horrible sights*, shrinking from them and avoiding to repair thither, and it is feared that sickness and manifold other harm will thereby arise to the friars and other of the people unless a speedy remedy be applied.[20]

That objections to slaughterhouses, piles of carrion and the like, so often refer to their unpleasant *appearance* as well as their disgusting smell was more than a simple question of aesthetics or affronted sensibilities.[21] As the rulers of Siena observed during a campaign to improve the inner city in the 1450s, the spectacle of butchers plying their trade in busy thoroughfares was not only incompatible with their drive for 'beautification and ornamentation', but also a serious risk to health.[22]

During the plague of 1368–1369 the 'abominable' and 'loathsome' sight of the carrion deposited in the streets by London butchers caused just as much alarm as did the ensuing 'corruption and grievous stench', resulting in the threat of imprisonment and a massive fine of £100 for offenders.[23] Once again, these measures were influenced by contemporary medical theory. According to the Islamic authorities who transmitted Aristotelian ideas about optics to the West, the eye was a passive organ which absorbed the impressions, 'forms', 'virtues', or 'similitudes' that radiated outwards in a continuous sequence of multiple images from all visible objects.[24] Late medieval physicians regarded the *aspectus*, or appearance, of rotting meat, overflowing gutters, and other visually offensive nuisances as a potential source of infection, warning that the 'species' of disease or physical decay might enter the eye of anyone who stared at them, eventually suffusing the entire venous system with corruption. Basic information along these lines had already reached the general populace by 1344, when one Scottish chronicler observed that, during an epidemic of poultry, 'men utterly shrank from eating, or *even looking upon* a cock or hen, as though unclean and smitten with leprosy'.[25]

Long recognised as a threat to survival, the consumption of contaminated meat seemed to pose an even greater risk during plague time because it, too, introduced toxins into the body. Responding in October 1348 to a royal commission of enquiry into the causes of the plague then raging throughout Europe, experts from the medical faculty of the University of Paris warned that individuals who failed to adopt 'a sensible and suitable dietary regimen' would automatically render themselves more susceptible to infection.[26] Their bodies might, in fact, be compared to dry kindling engulfed by a fire. In the 'nedefull and necessarie' vernacular treatise 'ayenst the pestilens' that he produced specifically for a 'lewde' readership during the plague-ridden 1470s, the Dominican Friar Thomas Multon adopted this powerful metaphor to explain in layman's terms why some people fell sick while others, who breathed the very same air, escaped unscathed:

> ye se wel and wete wel that the element of fire has non dominacion, ne wil not bren [burn] but in mater that is combustible and according [able] to receyue fire. On the same wise, the element of the aier that is pestilence corrupt infecte nother man, nother woman, ne childe, *but siche that hath venemes and corrupt humours within hemself.*[27]

On the one hand, the 'vnkyndely hete' generated during such a volcanic digestive process would open the pores, thereby allowing 'venomous ayere' easy access to the veins and arteries, while on the other the noxious matter arising from tainted food would make common cause with the invading miasmas as they advanced towards the heart.

Anxiety about the quality of the urban meat supply increased exponentially as patterns of consumption changed in the aftermath of the Black Death. Falling levels of population meant that the survivors enjoyed a far better and more carnivorous diet, with the result that the demand for meat, and especially beef, soared.[28] This, in turn, created a raft of problems for the authorities, not all of which might be immediately apparent today. There was, for instance, a dramatic rise in the number of butchers who faced prosecution for selling what appeared to be 'poisonable' or corrupt meat from bulls which had not been baited with dogs before slaughter. Drawing upon Galenic principles of physiology, contemporary opinion maintained that the 'violent heat and motion' of the tormented animal would convert 'utterly unwholesome' flesh and 'gross blood' into tender and nutritious meat.[29]

Whereas just two breaches of the relevant ordinance were reported by Ipswich jurors in 1438, the figure stood at five in 1465, eight in 1471 (the year of 'the most vnyuersall dethe' in living memory) and no fewer than eighteen in 1484, after a further sequence of devastating epidemics.[30] Such striking evidence, replicated in court records throughout England, testifies to a combination of mounting vigilance on the part of magistrates, of changing dietary habits and, most notably, of the spread of medical knowledge among the local communities which complained about such offences.

The level of concern demonstrated by urban authorities across the country is easy to understand when we consider the cumulative impact of plague epidemics during the late fourteenth and fifteenth century. Historians generally agree that following the national outbreaks of 1361–1362, 1368–1369, 1374–1345, and 1378–1379, plague became an increasingly local, and predominantly urban, phenomenon as its range, if not its virulence, decreased. But they have not always fully appreciated the long-term effects of this transition on communities already scarred by a dramatic fall in population and the economic, political, and social dislocation that so often followed. Major centres, such as Bristol, Coventry, Norwich, and York, were subject to recurrent, sometimes devastating attacks. Between 1400 and 1530, London alone experienced at least twenty-four localised outbreaks, together with thirteen national epidemics, averaging once every three and a half years, as was the case in Venice.[31] During the combined epidemic of sweating sickness and plague that swept the country in 1517, Sir Thomas More observed that 'one is safer on the battlefield than in the city', expressing in one neat epigram the siege mentality that had shaped generations of Londoners.[32] News of incipient epidemics occasioned acute anxiety since there was no means of telling how serious they might become. Predictably, those that did prove lethal tended to prompt a flurry of legislation, as well as a desire to enforce existing byelaws more effectively.

## Slaughterhouses, scalding houses, and meat markets

Urban authorities acknowledged four principal and interconnected areas of collective responsibility where the sanitary aspects of butchery were concerned. Sir Thomas More had already expressed firm opinions on the subject in his tale of the imaginary island of Utopia, which was notable for its extramural slaughterhouses where 'gore and offal' could be safely flushed away in streams and rivers, 'for fear that the air, tainted by putrefaction, should engender disease'.[33] With varying degrees of success, many English towns and cities had been investing for over a century in the provision of purpose-built facilities for slaughtering animals and preparing their carcasses away from major thoroughfares and central locations so that dung, carrion, and other refuse would pose less of an environmental hazard. Specialist flesh markets, where meat could be sold in hygienic conditions, might also be assigned to more peripheral areas, or at least to places which were easier to police. Then came the safe removal and disposal of noxious waste; and last, but not least, the enforcement of food standards through the regular scrutiny of the urban meat supply by salaried officials, local residents and, indeed, the butchers themselves.

Most English towns instigated some type of ban on the killing of animals in public places, and many went further by demanding the obligatory use of communal facilities, where butchers could work out of sight, without polluting neighbouring highways and gutters. In 1421 (a plague year) the rulers of Coventry proposed to construct an extramural scalding-house, warning that, once it was 'full fynyshid and redy', anyone who failed to use it would be liable for a substantial fine of 20*s* on each occasion.[34] In the meantime, they were, however, obliged to allow butchers to continue slaughtering animals on their own premises within the walls, on the condition that each of them kept 'his durre [doorway] clene fro bloode and other fylthis', and refrained from tethering or killing any animals in the street.[35] By the mid-fifteenth century, when the scalding-house was fully operational, with a permanent staff of four men appointed by the butchers' guild, it occasionally proved necessary to remind offenders of the penalty for non-compliance, but on the whole, the scheme appears to have worked well.[36]

The 1420s, a decade notable for localised epidemics, witnessed considerable activity in this respect, for it was then that the burgesses of Reading decided to invest heavily in the rebuilding and improvement of their 'scleynge house', which was equipped with a new well, stone flooring and a series of tiled gutters to facilitate cleansing.[37] Alarmed by the 'abomination, filth and *viliditatem putredorum*' of the 'rotting remains' in front of Butcher Row, Salisbury's magistrates decreed in 1423 that the slaughtering of animals should henceforth be relegated to the back, and that no offal should be carried away or fat rendered into tallow by day on account of the stench.[38] Some twenty years later, a former mayor himself erected a new 'skaldynghous' at his own cost, so that, as in Coventry, butchery could be restricted to one spot.[39] Similar rules concerning the use of designated premises obtained in Gloucester, largely to preserve the cleanliness of public thoroughfares.[40] The authorities also instituted special measures in 1514 (a year of 'great sickness') for the compulsory disposal of butchers' waste by night in order to avoid the 'inordinate savour and stynche that the comen gorreour [raker] makith by daye when he carieth awey innewardes of bestes, filthi vessels and other filthy thynges out of the Bocher Rewe'.[41] Arrangements of this kind, which were by then widespread, served to limit the circulation of contaminated air and offer residents some level of protection against the threat of infection.

Sanitary, as well as commercial considerations, also began to influence the location, layout, and facilities of the places where meat was on sale to the public. Well before the Black Death, larger towns and cities across Europe had invested in the creation of specialist meat markets, many of which now began to seem noisome and unhealthy. In 1416, the advisers of King Charles VI of France ordered the demolition of Paris's Great Butchery (Les Halles), which stood alarmingly near the royal palace of the Châtelet, and its replacement by four new flesh markets outside the walls. The adjacent slaughter- and scalding houses were likewise to be moved to a site beyond the Tuileries 'less dangerous to the public health of our said city and less likely to corrupt the air of the same'. The entire operation was justified on medical grounds, it being deemed necessary 'to provide and take precautions against the infections and corruptions noxious to the human body' (*pour pourveoir et obvier aux infections et corruptions nuisables a corps humain*) proceeding from such a filthy environment.[42] In the event, the Butchery was rebuilt on the same site along more spacious and hygienic lines, but the other provisions remained in force. Improvements of this kind were already underway in England, notably at London's Stocks market (see the map in Figure 1.1), which had originally been designed, in 1274, on the Parisian model.

It had taken almost seventy years to remove some of the more recalcitrant butchers of Cheapside from the streets and confine them to the Stocks area, as initially intended. By 1359, this imposing structure boasted seventy-one covered stalls or 'plots' arranged in wide parallel rows for vendors of meat and fish, and twenty-seven more beneath the pentices on the outer walls.[43] It is tempting to suggest that the decision to replace the market with an even more impressive three-storey stone structure half a century later was influenced by the medical advice supplied to the rulers of London during the devastating plague of 1407 (which was compared by one chronicler to Ovid's 'furnace blasts of death').[44] At all events, the new building was far easier to keep clean with flushing water from the nearby Walbrook (see the map in Figure 1.1); and we know from the accounts of the Bridge Wardens who managed it that significant sums were spent on the regular removal of noxious waste.[45] In Exeter, too, a sizeable investment was made during the early 1380s in the 'fleshfold', or meat market, which more than doubled in size to accommodate at least twenty-six butchers in a spacious, customised building that, like the Stocks, 'reflected the authorities' eagerness to guarantee the sale of quality meat and to curb sanitation hazards'.[46]

Being among the wealthiest, as well as the most tightly organised and heavily regulated, members of the late medieval victualling trades, the butchers themselves did not always welcome these initiatives, largely because some of the attendant costs might be passed on to them in the form of higher rents or service charges. This happened at Reading in 1459, when major structural changes were made to the above-mentioned slaughterhouse, resulting in a standoff between the authorities and the butchers, who refused to use it until the rent was reduced.[47] The dispute dragged on for at least five years and serves as another salutary reminder that financial interests could occasionally undermine the best-intentioned sanitary measures. Indeed, while generally – if sometimes reluctantly – accepting the need for more hygienic working practices, butchers were often intransigent in the face of external pressure, preferring to devise their own pragmatic solutions which would cause the least disruption.

## Waste disposal

The safe removal of carcasses, especially in hot weather, taxed the ingenuity of urban authorities to the limit and, as we have seen, might in extreme cases prompt royal intervention. Coastal towns and those situated on tidal or fast-flowing rivers had a ready means of disposal to hand, although butchers were inclined to cut corners by depositing their waste too close to the bank in residential areas where fresh water was essential for domestic consumption and in other inappropriate places. For this reason, designated dispersal points (such as the ironically named 'Douce Hill' and 'Le Balle', situated beside the Great Ouse to the north and south of King's Lynn)[48] were frequently set aside for compulsory use. Since contaminated water, and especially water that had been polluted with blood and offal, was regarded as a principal source of miasmatic air, it was vital that noisome matter should be flushed away as quickly and effectively as possible, preferably at ebb tide and in small pieces that would not block adjacent water gates, drains or gutters.[49]

Winchester's butchers clearly found it inconvenient to restrict their activities to the single site approved by the civic authorities in, or before, 1370 and stood accused of tipping entrails indiscriminately into the many watercourses that converged into the River Itchen. The cathedral monks (whose cemetery served as an illicit shortcut and general dumping ground) took particular exception to these insanitary practices. In 1398 they had to insert an iron grating across one particular stream to prevent 'dung, carcasses and entrails' from flooding into the neighbouring college; and a decade later they joined with other residents in demanding that all items of butchers' waste should be cut into segments no longer than four inches. The stipulation that any fines were to be raised, in the first instance, from the goods of the master of the craft was clearly effective and it proved unnecessary to repeat the ruling for over a century.[50]

The construction of piers or jetties from which processed waste could be thrown into deep water, well away from the river bank at ebb tide was another option, adopted first in York and then, more effectively, in London. Partly as a result of ongoing complaints by the Franciscans, in 1371 York's butchers were ordered by the civic authorities to build a pier that would extend into the Ouse well below the friary and to cease contaminating the water used by brewers and bakers with 'refuse of pigs or offal or any other noisome stuff'.[51] Since, as we have seen, the butchers evidently continued to litter the riverbank near their precinct with viscera, the Franciscans turned instead to King Edward, who imposed a draconian fine of 100s upon recidivists.[52] The mayor's decision to reduce the fine in line with civic custom hardly improved matters. Indeed, the survival of two further protests addressed by the friars to the Crown in 1380 and 1428 suggests that the authorities may have been more concerned to protect the environment in densely populated inner-city areas rather than prioritising the needs of religious houses on the urban periphery. On the other hand, they did take steps to make butchers' waste available for agricultural use by having it shipped out of the city by local farmers from a designated spot beside the river.[53]

Attempts to solve the problems experienced in London, especially with regard to waterborne pollution in the area around St. Nicholas Shambles, dragged on for over three decades largely because it proved impossible to find a viable solution that would satisfy all parties, including the Londoners who wanted cheap meat.

Finally, in 1393, a scheme was proposed for the compulsory removal of waste to Queenhithe on the Thames (see the map in Figure 1.1), where it could be processed and then conveyed in boats from a jetty to the centre of the river for disposal at ebb tide. A building, known as the 'puddynge house' or 'barrow house' was to be constructed there for dismembering carcasses, appropriately on the site of a former dunghill.[54] The scheme, which secured parliamentary approval, proved so successful that in 1402 the butchers of East Cheap secured a lease from the corporation of a lane leading to the river, where they built a bridge with houses upon it to serve a similar purpose.[55] Not until 1472 (a plague year) does the system appear to have broken down, evidently because the Thames had become so polluted with unprocessed offal that Edward IV was driven to protest.[56] Despite his intervention, the situation seems to have grown steadily worse. Having complained repeatedly to the civic authorities about the 'violence of unclene and putrified waters' flooding their streets, the disgruntled residents of the two parishes nearest St. Nicholas Shambles finally sought redress from parliament in 1488. Astutely warning that the king himself would be 'anoyde and invenemd by corrupt eyrs ingiendrid . . . by occacion of blod and other fouler thynges' whenever he came to worship at St. Paul's Cathedral, they managed to reintroduce the ban upon slaughtering within the walls of any English town that had obtained before 1393.[57]

St. Nicholas Shambles was, however, again in use by 1516, when Henry VIII, quite possibly at the instigation of Cardinal Wolsey, complained about it. At Wolsey's behest, a committee of aldermen was appointed two years later while plague was raging across England 'to choose at their discretion places outside the city where slaughterhouses might be made'.[58] The Cardinal and his physician, Thomas Linacre, had by then produced the first English quarantine regulations specifically for the containment of 'contagious infections', which were promulgated in London in January 1518, and were clearly determined to eliminate such an offensive and insanitary nuisance once and for all.[59] The prospect of a permanent return to the difficult situation that had obtained in the late fourteenth century clearly concentrated the butchers' minds. They decided to take pre-emptive action by embarking 'at theyr great and ymportunate costes and charges' upon the construction of a series of stone-lined 'wayes and vaultes under the grounde' that would carry all the polluted water and waste from St. Nicholas Shambles directly into the Thames. Formal permission, granted in 1532–1533 for slaughtering to resume within the walls was, significantly, conditional upon their readiness to undertake all the necessary 'scowryng, mayntenyng and kepyng of the vaultes', along with the speedy 'reformacion and amendment of all maner anoysances' that might subsequently ensue.[60]

As this protracted case so vividly reveals, one of the many challenges faced by urban butchers was the prompt and effective transportation of waste from slaughterhouse or market to the final point of disposal. It was common to fine or even imprison offenders who endangered others by littering streets, gardens, and yards with the 'annoyable' remains of butchered animals, but less easy to offer a viable alternative. Clearly influenced by the system already adopted in London, York's magistrates ruled during the national epidemic of 1378–1379 that any wagons used to carry offal to the River Ouse had always to be covered, in order to reduce airborne pollution as well as spillages.[61] The rulers of King's Lynn openly acknowledged their debt when, in 1439, they instructed all the resident butchers to equip themselves with 'covered wheelbarrows or carts according to the *regimen* adopted in London' or face a 20*s* fine.[62] Ten years later they added the further requirement that entrails and other unpleasant matter should only be conveyed through the town late in the evening or at daybreak when all law-abiding residents were safely indoors.[63] The repetition of local ordinances and the threat of exemplary (and in many cases unrealistic) fines suggests that it could sometimes be difficult to enforce measures of this kind, especially once the immediate threat of an epidemic had passed. In 1420, when plague hit Colchester, three-quarters of the town's resident butchers, who had grown casual about hygiene, were penalised for allowing offal to accumulate below their stalls and contaminate the air. Bad habits eventually returned, and between 1466 and 1474 many of them, including on one occasion the master of the craft himself, stood accused of failing adequately to maintain the carts in which they were supposed to transport waste beyond the walls.[64] Similarly, in 1504–1505 (another plague year) no fewer than eighteen of Chester's butchers incurred fines of 3*s* 4*d* each for slaughtering animals in their shops and throwing the detritus into the street. Prompt action evidently produced the desired effect, since no further charges seemed warranted.[65] Once it began to appear dangerous, laxity of this kind rapidly grew unacceptable, not only to urban magistrates but also to the local residents whose health was imperilled.

Of particular interest in this context is a lawsuit brought in the autumn term of 1450 in the King's Bench, England's premier criminal court, by Thomas Cornwaleys, the owner of a property just outside Aldgate (to the east of the Stocks market: see the map in Figure 1.1) against six London butchers. Claiming that he and his servants had already succumbed to a variety of ailments because the stench (*fetor*) of intestines and other vile matter dumped in his garden and outside his home had infected the air, he demanded crippling damages of £40. It was, he added, impossible for them to occupy the premises any longer without seriously endangering their health (*absque maximo corporum suorum periculo*). Significantly, after an initial delay the defendants were committed to prison just as plague reached Westminster in early December, being eventually released on bail provided by their fellow-butchers. The outcome of the case is now unknown, but it is clear that such allegations carried considerable weight and that litigants were well aware of the ways in which they could exploit current beliefs about environmental health to their advantage.[66]

In order to render their waste less immediately repugnant, butchers would also sink pits in which to safely bury the viscera and blood of animals or store them on a temporary basis, pending removal. From 1423 onward, any Coventry butcher failing to utilise 'the pitt vndur the Poody Croft' faced a fine of 4*d* for each offence.[67]

Fifteen years later the burgesses of Salisbury opted to dig a deep pit in the market so that piles of ordure and noxious remains would not contaminate the area around the stalls where food was on sale and people congregated.[68] As in the case of urban cesspits, the emptying process was so profoundly disagreeable that some communities deemed it necessary to regulate this activity, too. In Worcester, for example, a decree of 1466 established that:

> no entrails of any kind of beasts, nor any pits containing blood are to be cleansed or [the contents] carried away during the daytime, but only at night at an appropriate time . . . and that no pit containing blood should remain uncleansed for longer than one day and one night, be it winter or summer, on pain of 12*d* . . . as often and as many times as the offence is committed.[69]

## The quality of the urban meat supply

As a further offensive in their battle against plague, urban authorities sought to prevent the sale of any foodstuffs that would render consumers less able to resist the onslaught of toxic miasmas or that were themselves likely to pollute the air. Because of its propensity to deteriorate in warm weather, pork attracted particular scrutiny and its sale was often prohibited in summer. By the late fifteenth century Yarmouth butchers who dealt in contaminated meat 'to the grave peril and infection of the people' were liable to an exemplary fine of 20*s*, which was about fifteen times more than that currently imposed for assault.[70] Penalties of this size underscored the enormity of the offence, especially in a port that had suffered badly from successive epidemics of plague. Yet vigilance was universal. Again during the 1470s, Northampton's butchers were specifically required to establish the 'clennes' of every pig that they bought for slaughter by acquiring a formal 'warantise', or verbal guarantee, from the seller. No fewer than six of the fifty-eight byelaws then copied into the town's *Liber custumarium* concerned butchery, which was, not surprisingly, the most heavily regulated of all local crafts and trades.[71]

Food standards could be policed in three principal ways. By the later fifteenth century, if not before, many towns retained salaried inspectors, whose task was made easier by the construction of specialist meat markets or the creation of designated 'rows' where butchers were legally obliged to trade. By the 1480s, for example, 'flessh sayers' had been appointed in Leicester to patrol the shambles, their primary task being to examine all meat 'that it be not takket [spotted] with pok, moreyn, mesell [leprosy] ne non other contagyous syknes ne defaulte, but that it be gode, holsome and conuenient for mannys body'.[72] Ordinary residents were also encouraged to make complaints or 'presentments' for submission at regular intervals to local courts. Lists of the type of offences that merited investigation increasingly focused upon insanitary nuisances in general and butchers' misdemeanours in particular. One compiled in King's Lynn during the 1460s expected jurors to report:

alle bochers with in this towne that selle ony vnholsome fleshes, mesell [leprous] flesshe, raumes [rams'] fleshe, bulles fleshe vnbaited, roten moten, blowen flesshe, in deceite of the kynges people; and of alle bochers that slen [slaughter] ony bestes in the stretes or defoulen the stretes or the watir gates of this toun with blode, bones or entrailes of bestes [to] the noisance of the commones.[73]

Evidence of this kind not only reveals the ways in which basic concepts of health and hygiene were popularised, but also provides an important insight into collective involvement in the struggle against plague and the containment of hazardous behaviour.[74] Late medieval attempts to contain insanitary nuisances have been deemed inherently impractical because of their reliance on popular consensus, but there is good reason to suppose that peer pressure constituted a powerful inducement to compliance, at least when the urban body seemed to be under threat.[75]

Some of this pressure came from the butchers themselves, through the medium of their craft guilds, which oversaw working practices and had a vested interest in retaining public confidence. The involvement of these organisations in sanitary policing has hitherto received only limited attention and merits further study. The nuisances deemed ripe for inquiry by Colchester juries from the time of the 1375 plague onward not only included the sale of diseased or contaminated meat, but also any attempt to prevent 'the masters of the bochers craft' from performing 'there office wele and truly as they schuld do'.[76] In the highly regulated and protectionist environment of late medieval towns, such men exercised considerable power, not least with regard to the implementation of quality controls. In conjunction with civic officials, they were responsible for devising and enforcing appropriate ordinances for the government of their brethren, who had to comply, if necessary under threat of imprisonment or expulsion. Their visible presence was itself reassuring. Dressed 'in seemely apparrell and good arraye', from at least the late fifteenth century the warden of Exeter's butchers had to escort the mayor on a tour of the shambles every Saturday and report any 'defaults' at the guildhall on Mondays.[77] Delegation often proved necessary to cope with the amount of supervisory work involved. At the height of the 1479 plague epidemic, Lynn's butchers elected four of their number to inspect the goods on sale in the port's two busy meat markets, to collect the substantial fines imposed on offenders and to ensure that all waste was promptly removed in covered carts for disposal into the Great Ouse at ebb tide. The latter task, which also involved clearing away any offensive matter that had accumulated near the water gates, proved so onerous that in 1490 a weekly rota system was introduced, along with a substantial fine of 40*d* for anyone who missed his turn.[78]

Just six years earlier London's Company of Butchers had been empowered by the Court of Aldermen to inspect all boars and hogs brought into the city, to confiscate and destroy any found unwholesome and to report serial offenders to the authorities.[79] It was because of their vigilance that John Pynkard was caught selling four flitches of rancid bacon during the plague epidemic of 1517. Such a serious offence merited condign punishment. He was paraded along Cheapside from Newgate to Leadenhall market on horseback (see the map in Figure 1.1), with two of the flitches hung around his neck and the others carried in front of him. This motley procession included an official banging on a basin to attract the crowds, explaining to those who could not read the placard displayed above Pynkard's head that he had seriously endangered public health 'for puttyng to sale of mesell and stynkyng bacon'.[80]

These theatrical and highly ritualised spectacles were far from common, being generally confined to periods of acute dislocation, such as epidemics and attendant food shortages, when reliable meat supplies were hard to come by. Indeed, their relative rarity made them all the more dramatic, and the message they conveyed unusually forceful. Although they have in the past been cited out of context as evidence of the powerlessness of urban authorities to protect an ignorant public from disease, the evidence presented here would suggest the exact opposite. In the case of John Pynkard and William Brok, with whom this chapter began, we can detect a firm grasp of current medical ideas about infection and the transmission of disease, a desire to communicate this information to the wider public, and, above all, a coherent strategy for combating the miasmas of plague.

## Notes

1 Hudson (ed.), *Leet Jurisdiction in the City of Norwich*, 80. For the impact of plague on fourteenth-century Norwich see Rawcliffe, *Urban Bodies*, 14, 65–67, 70–71.
2 Sharpe (ed.), *Calendar of Letter-Books of the City of London, E*, 110–111; Riley (ed.), *Memorials of London*, 240–241; Jones, *Butchers of London*, 132; Rawcliffe, *Urban Bodies*, 264, note 181.
3 Cipolla, *Public Health and the Medical Profession*, 15. The same concerns were reiterated in 1501, when the Health Commissioners warned that rotten meat could 'infect this city with pestilential disease': Wheeler, 'Stench in Sixteenth-Century Venice', 27–28, 29–30.
4 Riley (ed.), *Memorials of London*, 312–313.
5 Sabine, 'Butchering in Mediaeval London', 342, 343.
6 Jones, *Butchers of London*, 80 and Chapter 4 generally.
7 Carr, 'Controlling the Butchers', 460. In her survey of regulations for the control of butchery and the sale of meat in medieval France, Madeleine Ferrières observes a connection between rules about hygiene enacted in the north after 1350 and '*la vague pesteuse*'. She does not, however, develop this point: *Histoire des peurs alimentaires*, 59 and Chapter 4 generally.
8 Geltner, 'Public Health and the Pre-Modern City', 231–245.
9 Benedictow, 'New Perspectives in Medieval Demography', 33. See also Bayless, *Sin and Filth in Medieval Culture*, 31.
10 For religious responses to, and scientific explanations of, plague see Horrox (ed.), *Black Death*, Chapters 3 and 4.
11 British Library, Additional MS 27582, fol. 71v.
12 Pickett, 'Translation of the "Canutus" Plague Treatise', 274. Beyond noting that 'smell and the disease that came along with it . . . significantly motivated regulations related to . . . butchery practices', Dolly Jørgensen makes no reference to this literature in her essay on 'The Medieval Sense of Smell', 309–312.
13 Avicenna, *Liber Canonis Medicine*, book IV, fol. 329r. This passage is cited almost verbatim in one of the earliest printed vernacular English plague tracts, Anon, *A Litill Boke Necessarye and Behouefull agenst the Pestilence*, n.p.

14  Rawcliffe, *Urban Bodies*, 45–52, 123–124.
15  Cooper (ed.), *Annals of Cambridge, I*, 114. These and other sanitary measures were prom- ulgated by local magistrates in response to complaints from the university.
16  Sabine, 'Butchering in Mediaeval London', 344–349; Riley (ed.), *Memorials of London*, 456–458; Jones, *Butchers of London*, 78–80. These disputes, some of which predated the Black Death, are also discussed by Rexroth, *Deviance and Power*, 103–107, in the context of civic ideals about 'purity' and the wider struggle of the authorities to contain a variety of other nuisances, including prostitution and mendicancy.
17  Given-Wilson *et al.* (eds.), *Parliament Rolls of Medieval England, VI*, 181. Such evidence undermines the contention that medieval responses to blood were largely dictated by ritual taboos rather than 'practical' (that is medical) considerations: Bildhauer, *Medieval Blood*, 66–67. Even so, some sense of blood as a pollutant survives in regulations of the kind in force at Henley, which made a particular point of protecting the high cross from defilement by butchers' waste: Briers (ed.), *Henley Borough Records*, 48, 142.
18  Luders *et al.* (eds), *Statutes of the Realm, Vol. 2*, 59–60. Higher levels of mortality may have been observed at the time in areas where unregulated butchery was carried out. During the 1400–1401 plague, one in four heads of household living in the Bourg area of Dijon, which was then notorious for its insanitary slaughterhouses, is known to have died: Galanaud *et al.*, 'Historical Epidemics Cartography'. I am grateful to Professor Galanaud for drawing my attention to his work.
19  The statute was widely publicised, being, for example, copied verbatim into the Oath Book of Colchester: Gurney Benham (ed.), *Oath Book*, 194–195.
20  *Calendar of Close Rolls, 1369–1374*, 438.
21  As assumed, for example, by Ciecieznski, 'Stench of Disease', 97.
22  Nevola, *Siena*, 97–98.
23  Thomas (ed.), *Calendar of Plea and Memoranda Rolls*, 93; *Calendar of Close Rolls, 1369–1374*, 31–32, 177–178. Sandwich's butchers were already by then forbidden from killing or eviscerating animals in public *view*, being required to perform such activities 'in a secret place': British Library, Cotton MS Julius B.IV, fol. 75v.
24  For the impact of these concepts on plague literature see Stearns, *Infectious Ideas*, 93–96.
25  Rawcliffe, *Leprosy in Medieval England*, 93–95.
26  Horrox (ed.), *Black Death*, 163.
27  British Library, Sloane MS 3489, fol. 45v.
28  Dyer, *Standards of Living*, 197–199, 199–202. In Colchester, for instance, the number of butchers rose from 13 in 1359 to 21 in 1400 (when the population stood at about 8,000). There were at least 20 by 1444, although numbers fell quite dramatically thereafter because of recession: Britnell, *Growth and Decline in Colchester*, 131, 199.
29  Luttrell, 'Baiting of Bulls and Boars', 23–24, 398–341.
30  Suffolk Record Office (Ipswich), C/2/8/1/11, 13, 20, C/2/10/1/2.
31  Rawcliffe, 'Introduction', 2.
32  Flood, '"Safer on the Battlefield than in the City"', 147.
33  More, *Utopia*, 138–139, 418.
34  Dormer Harris (ed.), *Coventry Leet Book, I*, 32. A labourer then earned about 4*d* a day, while 20*s* would have paid the annual rent on a large urban property.
35  *Ibid.*, 43. It was at this time that the King's Lynn authorities staged a crackdown on butchers who slaughtered animals in the streets, no fewer than thirteen of them, along with seven other householders, being fined for this offence in 1422 alone: King's Lynn Borough Archives, KL/C 17/13 (court leet re-dated from the reign of Richard II).
36  Dormer Harris, *Coventry Leet Book, I*, 232; *Ibid.*, *Coventry Leet Book, II*, 271, 279.
37  Slade (ed.), *Reading Gild Accounts 1357–1516, Part I*, lxxi–ii, 62–63, 68–69, 100–101, 106–109. The total cost, spread over seven years, came to over £13, which was more than double the annual income of the gild merchant that financed the rebuilding.
38  Carr (ed.), *First General Entry Book*, 236.
39  *Ibid.*, 398.
40  Stevenson, 'Records of the Corporation of Gloucester', 433, 440–441.

41  *Ibid.*, 440.

42  De Lespinasse (ed.), *Métiers et corporations de la ville de Paris*, 274.

43  Keene, *Walbrook Study*, 6; Rawcliffe, *Urban Bodies*, 263.

44  Rawcliffe, 'Introduction', 1, 6.

45  Keene, *Walbrook Study*, 6, 23, Figure 2; Sabine, 'Butchering in Mediaeval London', 341.

46  Kowaleski, *Local Markets*, 182–183, 188. The construction of large stone-built meat halls in Netherlandish towns and cities, such as Haarlem (1386), Ghent (1408) and Deventer (1414) is worth noting in this context: Coomans, 'In Pursuit of a Healthy City', 121.

47  Slade (ed.), *Reading Gild Accounts 1357–1516, Part II*, 44–47; Guilding (ed.), *Reading Records*, 58.

48  King's Lynn Borough Archives, KL/C 7/3, Hall Book, 1431–1450, fol. 103r. The rules were still often ignored. Again in 1422, thirteen Lynn butchers and twelve from the nearby village of Terrington were fined for disposing of offal and dung near the water gates: KL/C 17/13.

49  Rawcliffe, *Urban Bodies*, 188–197.

50  Keene, *Survey of Medieval Winchester*, 64; Bird (ed.), *Black Book of Winchester*, 18, 124.

51  Sellers (ed.), *York Memorandum Book, I*, lxvii, 15.

52  See above, note 20.

53  Sellers (ed.), *York Memorandum Book, I*, 17–18; *Calendar of Patent Rolls, 1377–1381*, 524; Sellers (ed.), *York Memorandum Book, II*, 70.

54  *Calendar of Close Rolls, 1392–1396*, 133; Sharpe (ed.), *Calendar of Letter Books of the City of London, H*, 372, 392; Jones, *Butchers of London*, 80, 82.

55  Sharpe (ed.), *Calendar of Letter-Books of the City of London, I*, 22.

56  *Ibid.*, *Calendar of Letter Books of the City of London, L*, 104.

57  Luders *et al.* (eds), *Statutes of the Realm, Vol. 2*, 527–528.

58  Jones, *Butchers of London*, 81.

59  Rawcliffe, *Urban Bodies*, 298. Wolsey's plans for Cardinal College, Oxford, paid predictable attention to hygiene. The slaughterhouse was to be 'cleansed with water, as oft as need shall require ... either by the common stream or else by policy': Salzman, *Building in England*, 411.

60  Luders *et al.* (eds), *Statutes of the Realm, Vol. 3*, 435.

61  Sellers (ed.), *York Memorandum Book, I*, lxix, 17–18.

62  Owen (ed.), *Making of King's Lynn*, 217. London butchers themselves occasionally needed reminding of these rules: Jones, *Butchers of London*, 80–81.

63  King's Lynn Borough Archives, KL/C 7/3, Hall Book, 1431–1450, fol. 271v.

64  Britnell, *Growth and Decline in Colchester*, 199–200, 202, 245.

65  Cheshire and Chester Archives and Local Studies Service, ZS/B/5b (Sheriffs' book, 1504–1505).

66  The National Archives, Kew, KB 27/758, rot. 51r. I am grateful to Dr Hannes Kleineke for drawing my attention to this case. For the 1450 plague, see Rawcliffe, *Urban Bodies*, 367–368.

67  Dormer Harris (ed.), *Coventry Leet Book, I*, 43. Significantly, in 1463 any butchers who wished to remain temporarily in central Siena (pending their permanent removal to custom-built suburban facilities) had to own a deep refuse well in which to store blood and viscera: Nevola, *Siena*, 97.

68  Carr (ed.), *First General Entry Book*, 163.

69  Smith and Smith (eds.), *English Gilds*, 385. The three previous years had witnessed outbreaks of plague.

70  Norfolk Record Office, Y/C4/186 (court leet 1481–1482), rot. 15r. A similar penalty was exacted in Coventry: Dormer Harris (ed.), *Coventry Leet Book, I*, 32.

71  Markham (ed.), *Records of the Borough of Northampton*, 226, 229–230. Each resident butcher also had to swear an oath that he would not sell 'any maner corupte fflessh' (*ibid.*, 395).

72  Bateson (ed.), *Records of the Borough of Leicester*, 321–322. In some Netherlandish towns, inspectors would place the confiscated rotten meat on a pole next to the stall

of the offender as a further warning to the public: Coomans, 'In Pursuit of a Healthy City', 117.
73 Norfolk Record Office, NCR, 5C/10. I am grateful to Ms Susan Maddock for drawing my attention to this document.
74 Rawcliffe, 'View from the Street'.
75 Jørgensen, 'Cooperative Sanitation', 566.
76 Gurney Benham (ed.), *Oath Book*, 2–4, 222–223.
77 Vowell *alias* Hooker, *Description of the Citie of Excester*, 818.
78 King's Lynn Borough Archives, KL/C 7/4, Hall Book, 1453–1497, 409, 530, 547, 574. For the epidemic see Rawcliffe, *Urban Bodies*, 370.
79 Sharpe (ed.), *Calendar of Letter Books of the City of London, L*, 216.
80 Jones, *Butchers of London*, 132–133.

# References

## Archival sources

British Library, Additional MS 27582; Cotton MS Julius B.IV; Sloane MS 3489.
Cheshire and Chester Archives and Local Studies Service, ZS/B/5b (Sheriffs' book, 1504–1505).
King's Lynn Borough Archives, KL/C 7/3, Hall Book, 1431–1450; KL/C 7/4, Hall Book, 1453–1497; KL/C 17/13 (court leet, 1422).
Norfolk Record Office, NCR, 5C/10; Y/C4/186 (court leet, 1481–1482).
Suffolk Record Office (Ipswich), C/2/8/1/11, 13, 20; C/2/10/1/2.
The National Archives, Kew, KB 27/758.

## Printed primary sources

Anon, *A Litill Boke Necessarye and Behouefull agenst the Pestilence* (London: W. de Machlinia, c. 1485).
Avicenna, *Liber Canonis Medicine* (Lyon: Jacques Myt, 1522).
Bateson, Mary (ed.), *Records of the Borough of Leicester, II* (London: CJ Clay and Sons, 1901).
Bird, W. H. B. (ed.), *The Black Book of Winchester* (Winchester: Warren and Son, 1925).
Briers, P. M. (ed.), *Henley Borough Records: Assembly Books I–IV, 1395–1543* (Banbury: Oxfordshire Record Society, 41, 1960).
*Calendar of Close Rolls, 1369–1374* (London: HMSO, 1911).
*Calendar of Close Rolls, 1392–1396* (London: HMSO, 1925).
*Calendar of Patent Rolls, 1377–1381* (London: HMSO, 1895).
Carr, David R. (ed.), *The First General Entry Book of the City of Salisbury 1387–1452* (Trowbridge: Wiltshire Record Society, 54, 2001).
Cooper, C. H. (ed.), *Annals of Cambridge, I* (Cambridge: Warwick & Co., 1842).
Dormer Harris, Mary (ed.), *The Coventry Leet Book, I* (London: Early English Text Society, original series, 134, 1907).
Dormer Harris, Mary (ed.), *The Coventry Leet Book, II* (London: Early English Text Society, original series, 135, 1908).
Given-Wilson, Christopher, Paul Brand, Seymour Phillips, Mark Ormrod, Geoffrey Martin, Anne Curry, and Rosemary Horrox (eds.), 'The Parliament Rolls of Medieval England, VI' (Woodbridge: Boydell Press, 2005).
Guilding, J. M. (ed.), *Reading Records: Diary of the Corporation I* (London: James Parker & Co., 1892).

Gurney Benham, William (ed.), *The Oath Book: or Red Parchment Book of Colchester* (Colchester: Essex County Standard Office, 1907).

Horrox, Rosemary (ed.), *The Black Death* (Manchester: Manchester University Press, 1994).

Hudson, William (ed.), *Leet Jurisdiction in the City of Norwich* (London: Selden Society, 5, 1891).

Lespinasse, René de (ed.), *Les métiers et corporations de la ville de Paris I: XIVe–XVIIIe siècle, ordonnances générales metiers de l'alimentation* (Paris: Imprimerie Nationale, 1886).

Luders, Andres, Thomas Edlyne Tomlins, John France, William Elias Taunton, and John Raithby (eds.), *Statutes of the Realm, 11 Vols* (London: Record Commission, 1810–1828).

Markham, C. A. (ed.), *The Records of the Borough of Northampton, I* (London: Elliot Stock, 1898).

More, Thomas, *Utopia*, in E. Surtz and J. H. Hexter (eds.), *The Complete Works of St. Thomas More, Volume 4* (New Haven, NJ: Yale University Press, 1965).

Owen, Dorothy M. (ed.), *The Making of King's Lynn: A Documentary Survey* (Oxford: Records of Social and Economic History, new series, 9, 1984).

Pickett, J. P. (ed.), 'A Translation of the "Canutus" Plague Treatise', in: Lister M. Matheson (ed.), *Popular and Practical Science of Medieval England* (East Lansing, MI: Medieval Texts and Studies, 11, 1994).

Riley, H. T. (ed.), *Memorials of London and London Life in the XIIIth, XIVth and XVth Centuries* (London: Longmans, Green & Co., 1868).

Sellers, Maud (ed.), *York Memorandum Book, I* (Durham, UK: Surtees Society, 120, 1912).

Sellers, Maud (ed.), *York Memorandum Book, II* (Durham, UK: Surtees Society, 125, 1915).

Sharpe, R. R. (ed.), *Calendar of Letter-Books of the City of London, E* (London: John Edward Francis, 1903).

Sharpe, R. R. (ed.), *Calendar of Letter-Books of the City of London, H* (London: John Edward Francis, 1907).

Sharpe, R. R. (ed.), *Calendar of Letter-Books of the City of London, I* (London: John Edward Francis, 1909).

Sharpe, R. R. (ed.), *Calendar of Letter-Books of the City of London, L* (London: John Edward Francis, 1912).

Slade, Cecil (ed.), *Reading Gild Accounts 1357–1516, Part I* (Reading: Berkshire Record Society, 6, 2002).

Slade, Cecil (ed.), *Reading Gild Accounts 1357–1516, Part II* (Reading: Berkshire Record Society, 7, 2002).

Smith, Toulmin and Lucy Toulmin Smith (eds.), *English Gilds* (London: Early English Text Society, original series, 40, 1892).

Thomas, A. H. (ed.), *Calendar of Plea and Memoranda Rolls of the City of London, 1364–1381* (Cambridge, UK: Cambridge University Press, 1929).

Vowell, Iohn, *alias* Hooker, 'Description of the Citie of Excester, Part III', W. J. Harte, J. W. Schopp, and H. Tapley-Soper (ed.) (Exeter: Devon and Cornwall Record Society, 14, 1919).

## Printed secondary sources

Bayless, Martha, *Sin and Filth in Medieval Culture* (New York: Routledge, 2012).

Benedictow, Ole, 'New Perspectives in Medieval Demography: The Medieval Demographic System', in: Mark Bailey and S. H. Rigby (eds.), *Town and Countryside in the Age of the Black Death* (Turnhout: Brepols, 2012).

Bildhauer, Bettina, *Medieval Blood* (Cardiff: University of Wales Press, 2006).

Britnell, Richard H., *Growth and Decline in Colchester, 1300–1525* (Cambridge, UK: Cambridge University Press, 1986).

Carr, David R., 'Controlling the Butchers in Late Medieval English Towns', *The Historian*, 70, 3 (2008), 450–461.

Ciecieznski, N. J., 'The Stench of Disease: Public Health and the Environment in Late Medieval English Towns and Cities', *Health, Culture and Society*, 4, 1 (2013), 92–104.

Cipolla, C. M., *Public Health and the Medical Profession in the Renaissance* (Cambridge, UK: Cambridge University Press, 1976).

Dyer, Christopher, *Standards of Living in the Later Middle Ages* (Cambridge, UK: Cambridge University Press, 1989).

Ferrières, Madeleine, *Histoire des peurs alimentaires du Moyen Âge à l'aube du XXe siècle* (Paris: Éditions du Seuil, 2002).

Flood, J. L., '"Safer on the Battlefield than in the City": England, the "Sweating Sickness" and the Continent', *Renaissance Studies*, 17, 2 (2003), 147–176.

Geltner, G., 'Public Health and the Pre-Modern City: A Research Agenda', *History Compass*, 10, 3 (2012), 231–245.

Jones, P. E., *The Butchers of London* (London: Secker and Warburg, 1976).

Jørgensen, Dolly, 'Cooperative Sanitation: Managing Streets and Gutters in Late Medieval England and Scandinavia', *Technology and Culture*, 49, 3 (2008), 547–567.

Jørgensen, Dolly, 'The Medieval Sense of Smell, Stench and Sanitation', in: R. Beck, U. Krampl, and E. Retaillaud-Bajac (eds.), *Les cinq sens dans la ville du Moyen Âge à nos jours* (Tours: Presses Universitaires François-Rabelais, 2013), 301–313.

Keene, Derek, *Survey of Medieval Winchester, I* (Oxford: Winchester Studies, 2, 1985).

Keene, Derek, *The Walbrook Study: A Summary Report* (London: Institute of Historical Research, 1987).

Kowaleski, Maryanne, *Local Markets and Regional Trade in Medieval Exeter* (Cambridge: Cambridge University Press, 1995).

Luttrell, C. A., 'Baiting of Bulls and Boars in the Middle English "Cleanness"', *Notes and Queries*, 197, 2 (1952), 23–24; and 201 (1956), 398–341.

Nevola, Fabrizio, *Siena: Constructing the Renaissance City* (New Haven, NJ: Yale University Press, 2007).

Rawcliffe, Carole, 'Introduction', in: Linda Clark and Carole Rawcliffe (eds.), *Society in an Age of Plague* (Woodbridge: The Fifteenth Century, 2013), 1–14.

Rawcliffe, Carole, *Leprosy in Medieval England* (Woodbridge: Boydell Press, 2006).

Rawcliffe, Carole, 'The View from the Street: The Records of Hundred and Leet Courts as a Source for Sanitary Policing in Late Medieval English Towns', in: Carole Rawcliffe and Claire Weeda (eds.), *Policing the Environment in Premodern Europe* (Amsterdam: Amsterdam University Press, forthcoming, 2018).

Rawcliffe, Carole, *Urban Bodies: Communal Health in Late Medieval English Towns and Cities* (Woodbridge: Boydell Press, 2013).

Rexroth, Frank, *Deviance and Power in Late Medieval London*, Pamela E. Selwyn (trans.) (Cambridge, UK: Cambridge University Press, 2007).

Sabine, E. L., 'Butchering in Mediaeval London', *Speculum*, 8, 3 (1933), 335–353.

Salzman, L. F., *Building in England Down to 1540* (Oxford: Clarendon Press, 1967).

Stearns, Justin K., *Infectious Ideas: Contagion in Premodern Islamic and Christian Thought in the Western Mediterranean* (Baltimore: Johns Hopkins University Press, 2011).

Stevenson, William H., 'The Records of the Corporation of Gloucester', *Historical Manuscripts Commission Twelfth Report, Appendix, Part IX* (London: HMSO, 1891).

Wheeler, Jo, 'Stench in Sixteenth-Century Venice', in: A. Cowan and J. Steward (eds.), *The City and the Senses: Urban Culture since 1500* (Aldershot: Ashgate, 2006), 25–38.

## Electronic resources

Galanaud, Pierre, Anne Galanaud, and Patrick Giraudoux, 'Historical Epidemics Cartography Generated by Spatial Analysis: Mapping the Heterogeneity of Three Medieval "Plagues" in Dijon': https://journals.plos.org/plosone/article?id=10.1371/journal.pone0143866.

## Unpublished thesis

Coomans, J., 'In Pursuit of a Healthy City: Sanitation and the Common Good in the Late Medieval Low Countries' (PhD thesis, University of Amsterdam, 2018).

# 2

# PLAGUE IN EARLY MODERN LONDON

## Chronologies, localities, and environments[1]

*Vanessa Harding*

Plague was a fact of London life for more than three centuries. After its initial devastating impact in 1348–1351, in which a third to a half of London's population may have died, and two or three returns before 1400, its epidemiology and impact seem to have changed to a pattern of periodic, but less severe outbreaks through the fifteenth and early sixteenth centuries. From the mid-sixteenth century, when London itself was growing rapidly, plague epidemics are better documented, but also it seems more deadly, killing up to one-sixth or more of the population, though without sapping London's overall growth.[2] Over the period 1563–1665, perhaps 200,000 people died of plague in London, accounting for up to one-sixth of all deaths; there were five major epidemics, one less severe, and several periods of raised plague mortality.[3] After the 1665 epidemic, plague effectively disappeared from London, and the disease gradually retreated from Europe.[4]

Although early modern plague has been the focus of many studies, there still remain inconsistencies and puzzling elements in an apparently widely-accepted narrative. The identity of the pathogen or pathogens responsible for these thousands of deaths is still questioned. The severity of epidemics varied apparently randomly from episode to episode and from area to area, and patterns of incidence were inconsistent: while plague sometimes disappeared after a single terrible year, on two or three occasions it lingered for several years, killing a significant number over several consecutive years, but never flaring into a city-wide epidemic. Furthermore, although the quality and healthfulness of London's built environment, and arguably the general health and nutritional status of its population, deteriorated over the period, plague epidemics did not get successively worse in relation to population size.

In terms of elucidating the history of plague in London, there has been a tendency for historians to concentrate on the major epidemics or 'plague years' – the Bills of Mortality, a key source for the study of plague, were first compiled in and for plague years, and later writers and collectors of data tended to extract plague data and ignore the background. The major epidemics had a dramatic social as well as demographic impact and prompted outpourings of popular and learned publications. There is a strong focus also on the seventeenth-century plagues, especially that of 1665, though F. P. Wilson's *The Plague in Shakespeare's London* covers a key period and Paul Slack's study extends more widely; Graham Twigg's recent study also takes a broader view.[5] The mid- and early sixteenth-century epidemics, however, have been much less studied, though both Creighton and Shrewsbury at least covered the ground.[6] Fifteenth-century plagues are still less explored, though the fourteenth-century Black Death is well covered.[7] The historiographical break in the study of plague in London between the medieval and the early modern periods is caused partly by a change in the documentary sources available – parish registers begin in 1538, and only survive in quantity from *c.* 1558 – and partly simply by the tendency for medieval and early modern studies to separate around 1500–1550. Ultimately, a full understanding of plague and its impact on London will require an approach that integrates medieval and early modern evidence, local and national stories, and a wide geographical perspective.

A second problem has been what might be termed biological determinism: confidence that the disease early modern people called plague was identical with modern bubonic plague, responsible for the Third Pandemic, and therefore dependent on rats and fleas for its transmission.[8] This belief has shaped twentieth-century accounts of pre-modern plague's appearance, transmission, and eventual disappearance,[9] and particularly assessments of the efficacy of public health measures, and of steps to prevent or treat the disease.[10] Challenge to this identification dates back at least to Graham Twigg's 1984 study, *The Black Death: A Biological Reappraisal.*[11] It took longer for the implications of his argument, and the findings of studies of plague in continental Europe, to inform the study of early modern English plague, but most writers are now cautious about extrapolating from what is known of modern bubonic plague to draw conclusions about past phenomena.[12] Radical alternatives to the conventional diagnosis have been proposed; if no general consensus has yet been reached on the detail, it is at least acknowledged that the characteristics of early modern plague differ in many respects from modern bubonic plague.[13]

The aim of this chapter is to (re)consider plague in early modern London both as chronology and geography, and convey its complexity to an audience with a wider interest in the disease. There was not one plague but a succession of epidemics; not one geographical pattern but a shifting one. Underlying patterns of mortality and their change over time are crucial to an appreciation of the disease, and comparison of epidemic experiences at different periods may be useful. Approaches other than the epidemiological, however, still offer important insights into the experience of plague and how it was perceived by contemporaries. The chapter begins with an account of the official response to plague in the forms of data collection – the Bills of Mortality, which also provide a major source for charting plague's incidence in time and space – and attempts at control, by issuing Plague Orders and other directions, which help to reveal their understanding of the disease and its causes. The chapter then considers the broader chronology of plague incidence in early modern London, setting the epidemic years in context and reviewing available figures for mortality levels. The chronology of plague outbreaks links with the evidence for its geography, and prompts consideration of London's built environment and its relationship to plague mortality; possible environmental correlations are a key theme of the chapter. Although the chapter does not focus on the biological identity and epidemiology of early modern plague, and makes no assumptions on the subject, the evidence for Londoners' perceptions and experiences of plague contributes to a more accurate description of the disease, and the question of its identity is reviewed in a final section.

## Public authority and official responses

Over the sixteenth century, attempts to document plague mortality on a systematic basis, intended originally to inform authorities, evolved into the weekly Bills of Mortality, summaries of deaths and plague deaths by parish published as broadsides or handbills. By the seventeenth century the published Bills had become a regular feature of London life. They were compiled by the Parish Clerks' Company from returns from individual parishes, and printed under strict protocols to ensure that information went first to the Crown and Privy Council, and to the city of London. Their format was fixed, and considerable care was taken to ensure that no errors crept in, given the impact of the weekly figures and their distribution on confidence, morale, and indeed commerce. They were an important element in the government's response to plague, and informed action at a number of different levels. At its simplest, the justification for collecting the information on a regular basis was to be able to detect the onset of an epidemic – a sustained rise in weekly death totals in the early summer was a pretty good indication – so that those with responsibilities could plan their strategies.[14] A warrant of 1604 prescribed that theatres should close if the weekly total of plague deaths (which could only be generally known from the Bills) reached thirty. The threshold was revised upwards to forty in 1608, and remained at that level until 1642, though it seems as if the city often ordered the theatres closed before this level was reached.[15] John Graunt observed in 1662 that people read the weekly Bills to see

> how the Burials increase, or decrease; . . . and withall, in the Plague-time, how the Sickness increased, or decreased, that so the Rich might judge of the necessity of their removall, and Trades-men might conjecture what doings they were like to have in their respective dealings.[16]

In appearance and format the Bills evolved over time, but gradually became standardised as a highly-recognisable and legible genre. Serious as their content was, they were also works of conscious typographical design. Through their arrangement and presentation, they gave visual expression to the city's topography, listing the parishes in groupings that impressed a view of the metropolis as concentric, with a heart or core (the ninety-seven parishes within the walls) and peripheries (the sixteen parishes outside the walls, but wholly or partly within the city; the outparishes in Middlesex and Surrey). They made these groupings and the names of London parishes better known to residents and provincial correspondents alike.[17] The multiplicity of London's parishes also added finer grain to the overall information of the weekly Bills, enabling Londoners to monitor the spread of plague, to track the weekly progress of an epidemic across the city, and to identify and avoid infected parishes.[18]

By promoting the simple binary of deaths and plague deaths in columns for each parish, and in totals for different areas of the metropolis, the weekly Bills promoted a view of plague as a single, identifiable disease, with a strong spatial dimension. Although other causes of death were collected and came to be listed on the verso of the Bill, no other disease was given this prominence, or this spatial specificity: the 'Diseases and casualties' were reported for London as a whole. Yearly Bills were compiled from the weekly totals and both reiterated the variety of local experiences and contributed to a sense of the historic sweep of plague. Individual 'plague years' could be identified, and the figures from one epidemic compared with another. A sub-genre of composite or commemorative Bills developed from 1625 or earlier, published in plague years, charting the course of the current epidemic with weekly mortality totals to date, and often reprinting mortality figures from earlier plague years. Some of these, published during the epidemic, left blank spaces for readers to fill in successive weekly figures. These composite Bills also often conveyed advice, remedies or preventatives, and appropriate prayers, so the Londoner who read one gained information for immediate use along with material for reflection.[19]

The city had a coherent and on its own terms rational response to plague, an emergency plan activated when an epidemic seemed imminent, which again emphasised plague's unitary identity and fixed characteristics. The Plague Orders derived from the Crown and Privy Council, and were informed by medical thinking including continental practice,[20] but they were imposed and enforced by the city authorities. The broad principles and provisions of the Orders had been established by the end of the sixteenth century, and covered points such as a survey of 'visited' or infected houses; twenty-eight-day quarantine of infected houses and their occupants; destruction of clothes and household stuff from infected houses; street cleaning; killing stray dogs; searching or inspecting of all dead to determine the cause of death; and restriction of assemblies, including public burials and stage plays. Bodies were to be buried 6 ft (1.8m) deep, though there was no general restriction on burial inside churches.[21] Plague Orders were issued first as proclamations and later, it appears, as multi-page books or booklets, printed by the King's or the city's printer.[22] Some of the text and provisions varied over time, but the core prescriptions remained the same. Although they formed the basis of the official response to plague, it is clear that the Orders were not always effectively enforced. Nor did they cover every eventuality: there was a stream of further proclamations in plague years, exhorting observation of the Orders and adding new instructions.[23]

Minutes of the Court of Aldermen document other activities, including the appointment of physicians and surgeons, dealing with the city's pesthouses, and sporadic efforts to solve the city's burial problem.[24]

One of the most ubiquitous textual manifestations of plague was the labelling of infected houses. The 1583 Orders required a paper with the words *Lord have mercy upon us* to be put up over the door of infected houses, which was not to be defaced or taken down.[25] By 1665 this had been elaborated into the requirement

> that every House visited, be marked with a Red Cross of a foot long, in the middle of the door, evident to be seen, and with these usual Printed words, that is to say, *Lord have mercy upon us*, to be set close over the same Cross, there to continue until lawful opening of the same House.[26]

The image of the plague cross, and the phrase 'Lord have Mercy upon us', became fixed in popular understanding and discourse of the plague. Although 7 June 1665 was probably the first time the adult Samuel Pepys, born in 1633, had ever seen 'two or three houses marked with a red cross upon the doors, and "Lord have mercy upon us" writ there', he had no doubt what this 'sad sight' meant.[27]

The Plague Orders and the city's other activities give a good idea of official thinking about the disease. It is clear that they believed that infection could be passed from person to person, and that those who had had contact with the diseased (or with the dead) could themselves infect others either before or without succumbing to the disease themselves. Quarantining the sick or potentially sick was therefore believed to be vital, and shutting-up of houses, though controversial and certainly resisted, remained a key element in the city's strategy.[28] Congregations of people were to be avoided. Likewise, the clothing and bedding of the sick were a lingering potential source of infection and must be treated with care or preferably destroyed; certainly they were not to be allowed to circulate as before. Hackney coaches used to convey the sick to the pesthouse or elsewhere were to be aired and not used again for six days. Some broader environmental concerns were addressed: dirt and rubbish in the streets could infect the air, so householders were required to clean in front of their houses and rakers appointed to remove the waste. 'No Hogs, Dogs, or Cats, or tame Pigeons, or Conies' were to be kept in the city. It appears also that food quality might be implicated, in the form of 'stinking Fish, or unwholesome Flesh, or musty Corn, or other corrupt fruits', though it is not clear if the danger lay in their consumption, or merely in their presence (see also Rawcliffe above).[29] An official publication of 1636 added advice from the College of Physicians on fumigation for houses and churches and perfume and pomanders for the person.[30]

The College of Physicians remained the official source of medical advice and prescription, though by 1665 the traditional, Galenic, humoural understanding of disease they favoured had come under sustained attack from the newer 'Chemical', Paracelsian and Helmontian physicians. Galenic physicians largely saw the problem as one of internal balance and resistance to disease at the level of the individual;

the unpredictable incidence of plague, taking some and sparing others, even in the same household, seemed to support this view. The Physicians' prescriptions in 1636 recommended consuming foods that would 'resist putrefaction', and added a list of cordials, purges, vomits, and electuaries, both to guard against taking infection and to expel it if it had entered the body.[31] While these were largely personal preventives and remedies, the anonymous *Directions for the Prevention and Cure of the Plague, Fitted for the Poorer Sort*, published in 1665, aimed at more general application. A short six-page pamphlet, this offered homely advice on diet ('abstain from the boiled herbs of Colliflowers, Cabbage, Coleworts, Spinage, and Beets') and some inexpensive remedies drawn from the Galenic pharmacopoeia. Although not an official publication, it has some sense of speaking for authority, as its instructions and advice are very much in line with the Plague Orders (several of its recommendations are mandated there) and with civic regulations for the behaviour of the poor.[32]

The government of London has often been criticised for its handling of plague, both at the time and since. Regulation was limited and late; professional involvement was low; inertia blocked radical solutions. The Crown, rather than the city, took the lead. This is partly justified, but partly unfair. The city government did adopt and issue plague regulations, and certainly acknowledged the severity of the crises. Criticism came from both directions: from above for not doing enough; from below, for heavy-handedly imposing policies of human quarantine and trade embargo to the damage of the population. In practice, the city authorities supported a regulatory framework that passed much of the day-to-day burden to the parishes, the natural locus of care and support, but they also made city-wide collections and distributions of resources, and took some part in organising relief burial grounds when the parishes were no longer able to cope.[33]

Many of the official prescriptions were somewhat ambivalent about the source of plague danger, which could have been as much moral as epidemiological, and indeed most explanations acknowledged divine or supernatural origins as first causes.[34] The view that gatherings of people – especially at theatres and entertainments – were dangerous and must be curbed was not limited to epidemics, but the Plague Orders singled out for prohibition 'Playes, Bear-baitings, Games, Singing of Ballads, Buckler-play, or such like causes of Assemblies of people', and playing at the London theatres was suspended on numerous occasions.[35] 'Disorderly Tipling in Taverns, Alehouses, Coffee-houses and Cellars' was said to be 'the common Sin of this time, and greatest occasion of dispersing the Plague'.[36] Taverns and alehouses were not closed down, but a 9 o'clock curfew was imposed. 'The multitude of Rogues and wandering Beggers that swarm in every place about the City' were seen as 'a great cause of the spreading of the Infection', requiring to be cleansed or controlled.[37] If sin was in part the cause, then the remedy included repentance and penance. Fasting, prayers, and sermons, while not specified in the Plague Orders, were among the first measures imposed by authority. The disappearance of plague was likewise marked by official sermons of thanksgiving, drawing moral lessons and warnings.[38]

## Chronologies and geographies of plague

The format of the Bills of Mortality highlights the distinctive geography of plague, with local variations in incidence, and their long-period coverage also brings out change over time. Setting variation or change in context, however, often needs complementary material, to which London's parish records make a major contribution. They also go back further in time than the surviving Bills. Other sources, such as tithe and tax assessments, yield data for the comparison of parish population size, and the localisation of wealth and poverty.

The historiography of plague in early modern London is extensive, but three studies, in particular, have illuminated the interaction of geography and chronology. Paul Slack's *The Impact of Plague on Tudor and Stuart England* (1985) is a crucial work.[39] He was the first of modern writers on plague to take a broad view and to relate plague to social reactions and consequences. In an era before the wide availability of digitised and online data, he undertook an heroic reconstruction of mortality data for the city of London, using a sample of parish registers from 1538 and tracing annual totals of London will probates back to the fifteenth century. He facilitated contextualisation and comparison by calculating Crisis Mortality Ratios, comparing mortality in plague years with mortality in preceding years, thereby avoiding the problem that not all plague deaths were necessarily recorded as such. He was able to compare the severity of different epidemics, and the local severity of individual epidemics. His overview of long-term geographical and mortality patterns produced the important conclusion that the expected 'topographical bias in the distribution of mortality . . . was not obvious at all' in 1563, when deaths appeared to be concentrated in the wealthier city centre, but that there was a marked shift in the focus of plague from the city centre to suburbs, to a significant degree by 1603 and almost completely by 1665.[40] His conclusions were, however, limited to the city parishes, which by 1665 probably contained only half or less of the total population of the metropolis, and by the fact that only some fifty-six of these parishes (of 113 in all) had adequate surviving burial registers for the period.

Ten years later, and thanks to a funded research project and greater statistical resources, Justin Champion published *London's Dreaded Visitation: The Social Geography of the Great Plague in 1665*.[41] This narrowed the focus to one epidemic only, but extended the geographical range of study to include London's suburban parishes, and brought in data from the hearth tax returns of the early 1660s for comparison. His principal demographic source for broad comparison was the Bills of Mortality, but close analysis of several individual parishes drew on other local sources. He asked a range of important and interesting questions in relation to the epidemiology and incidence of the 1665 epidemic: everything from coincident disease crises to seasonality to clustering. The study is helpfully free from epidemiological preconception, a vital point given the developing scepticism of traditional ascriptions of the Second Pandemic purely to rat- and flea-borne bubonic plague. Key elements of the work are the correlation of social and economic data with mortality data, and especially the resultant maps of endemic as well as epidemic patterns of mortality. Champion's results complicate Slack's picture by showing different patterns of mortality in the inner and outer suburbs, and between the city and Westminster; he concludes that in 1665 the suburbs suffered a more 'violent' shock than the city and Westminster.

More recently, Neil Cummins, Morgan Kelly, and Cormac Ó Gráda's project on living standards and plague in London took advantage of data-mining techniques and the availability online of almost all of London's parish registers 'to reconstruct the spatial and temporal patterns of birth and death in London from 1560 to 1665'.[42] Their study covers the whole of the metropolis, 130 parishes north and south of the river, the majority of which have some surviving registers for the period, and their dataset includes the records of some 930,000 burials and 630,000 baptisms. Metaphorically also they cover a great deal of ground, considering the relative magnitude of different epidemics, the diffusion and seasonality of plague deaths, and the social geography of plague. Their collection and analysis of data for the sixteenth century is particularly useful. Their data overall support Slack's observation of the shifting intensity of plague from the city within the walls to the extramural and suburban parishes. Important conclusions on the overall geography of plague are that epidemics most often began in the north or north-eastern parishes and thereafter spread to the inner city; there is little or no evidence of epidemics originating in the dock areas along the Thames east of the city.

These three studies establish a detailed and convincing picture of the absolute and relative severity of early modern plague epidemics and in broad terms their geographical incidence and how this changed over time. Several aspects deserve further attention, however, notably the chronology and geography of plague outside epidemic years; the intersecting chronologies and seasonalities of plague and other diseases; and the possible relationship between environment and the incidence of plague.

## Chronology and incidence

The last century of plague in England (1563–1665) is the best recorded, but the disease had been present since the Black Death of 1348–1350.[43] For the period before the inception of parochial registration of vital events in 1538 we are reliant on chronicle evidence, the replacement of manorial tenants or ecclesiastical incumbents, and (with caution) on fluctuations in will probates, to identify epidemic years, even if causes cannot be determined. However, these sources will usually only be sensitive to larger-scale events, and endemic or underlying patterns remain hard to detect. The focus on bubonic plague also means that other diseases, such as the sweat and influenza, may be neglected, even though the influenza epidemic of the later 1550s was probably the single most severe disease episode of the early modern period.[44]

Drawing on will probates and chronicle evidence, Paul Slack points to frequent mortality crises associated with plague between 1498 and 1521, and suggests that 'plague was probably more common in the early sixteenth century than in the early seventeenth'.[45] Once parish register data – even if very patchy – are available, a clearer picture of year-to-year variation emerges. There is evidence for epidemics in London in 1548, 1563, 1578, the early 1580s, and 1592–1593.[46] The scale of 1548 is shadowy since only about thirty-five parish registers survive for that date, but another thirty registers begin between 1550 and 1563, and together these indicate that the epidemic of 1563 was one of the more severe of the whole period. Several parish registers report plague deaths as such in 1563, and some note the beginning or end of the epidemic; in others, a significant elevation of deaths above the norm tells the story.[47]

A complicating factor in charting plague mortality in the late sixteenth century is the circulation in print of contemporary figures which may not stand up to closer examination. John Stow's *Summarie of Englyshe Chronicles* (1565) gives total deaths for the (modern) calendar year 1563 for the 'Cytie and liberties thereof (conteining.108 parishes)' from all causes at 20,372, with 17,404 of plague; in 'the out parishes adioyning to the same Citie, being xi. Paryshes', 3,288 died of all causes and 2,732 of plague. In total, 23,660 died in all, and 20,136 of plague.[48] These figures have been widely accepted and cited, but caution is needed. Stow does not name his authority, but his figures agree so closely with the totals in a sixteenth-century manuscript memorandum in the Folger Shakespeare Library that they must share a common source.[49] However, examination of the parish-by-parish figures in the Folger manuscript indicates that while some are plausible, correlating with those in surviving parish registers, others are significantly greater than those in the relevant parish register, while a few are much lower.[50] Overall, the reported totals could exaggerate the actual totals by up to 10 per cent, thus challenging Sutherland's view that 1563 was possibly the most deadly, in relation to London's size, of any early modern plague epidemic.[51] Though undoubtedly severe, the status of the 1563 epidemic as 'the great plague' should probably be downgraded, and this concurs with Cummins, Kelly, and Ó Gráda's recent conclusion, on the basis of aggregated parish register data, that 'the plagues of 1563, 1603, 1625, and 1665 were all of roughly equal relative magnitude'.[52] 1563 is still nevertheless remarkable as the last major epidemic in which so many plague deaths (it appears) took place within the walls.

Whatever its mortality, the plague of 1563 effectively ended in mid-winter 1563–1564. The parish register of St. George Botolph Lane notes that 'the plague seast' after 26 January 1564,[53] and the figures in John Stow's *Historical Memoranda* suggest that there was little tail-over of plague mortality into 1564: ninety-five died of plague in January 1564, seventy-six in February, twenty-nine in March. Twenty-five deaths from plague were reported for the rest of 1564, one in 1565, and six in 1566.[54]

Cummins, Kelly, and Ó Gráda's chart suggests some year-to-year variation in total mortality over the next three decades, to *c*. 1592, with no dramatic peaks but quite high mortality in 1578 and 1582.[55] Surviving weekly totals from 1578 show that 3,568 died of plague out of a total of 7,830 deaths, with deaths building up from August and peaking in early October.[56] The 1580s seem to have seen irregular short cycles of elevated mortality, in which plague played some part.[57] A surviving printed text from 1582 states that over 3,000 died of plague that year in the city and outparishes, perhaps 2–3 per cent of the population. If these figures can be relied on, the outbreak appears to have centred on Southwark (548 plague deaths from the four reporting parishes) and to some extent the western inner suburbs, St. Bride (124), St. Sepulchre (362), and St. Andrew Holborn (89), though there were only 239 plague deaths in 'the out-parishes', presumably including the Westminster parishes. Of the 109 listed parishes in the city and Liberties, only four were clear of plague, but nineteen recorded three plague deaths or fewer.[58] Some parish registers indicate excess mortality in August and September of that year, but the register of St. Michael Cornhill notes 'The beginning of the plague' on 24 October, with a further fourteen plague deaths before the end of the year.[59] Several parishes also record plague deaths in 1581 and/or through 1583, in most cases with a late summer peak.[60]

Both 1592 and 1593 were epidemic years, but the figures given by different sources (most of them far from contemporary) vary.[61] How and why these conflicting figures came into being cannot all be explained, but the overall picture is again resolved by Cummins, Kelly, and Ó Gráda, whose aggregation of totals from parish registers shows that while total mortality in 1592 was over 9,000, a significant excess over expected mortality, 1593 was much more severe, with mortality from all causes nearing 20,000.[62] Only study of individual parishes, however, will show whether and where mortality was localised in 1592 or 1593. Significant local variation seems likely. In both St. Martin in the Fields and St. Botolph Aldgate, for example, at either end of the metropolis, mortality in 1592 was 1.6 times the average over the preceding five years, with both reporting some plague deaths from August onwards, whereas in 1593, mortality in St. Martin was 3.2 times the average, but in St. Botolph, 6.2.[63]

London experienced other severe problems in the mid-1590s, but plague was not it seems among them.[64] 1603, however, was another plague year. Concern about plague in Southwark in March and April was followed by more widespread infection in the city and Liberties north of the river, to the extent that the celebrations for King James's arrival and coronation largely bypassed the city.[65] In July, before the coronation, the letter-writer John Chamberlain noted that 'the sicknes increseth so fast upon us' that he determined to 'make all the hast I can out of towne, for yt growes hot here'.[66] Others, sick and well, evidently fled likewise.[67] The emptying-out of the wealthier sort had a marked impact on the topography of mortality, with parishes in the centre of the walled city, badly hit in 1563, now much less severely affected, while parishes just inside and just outside the wall returned much higher figures than before.[68] Weekly death totals increased sharply from mid-July, and total deaths had reached 32,353, with 27,710 of plague, by early October. Figures for the whole year approached 40,000, with over 30,000 dying of plague.[69]

From 1604 onwards, though original yearly Bills of Mortality only survive sporadically, annual totals of deaths and plague deaths in the Bills are summarised by Graunt, and form the basis for many of his analyses and observations. The epidemic of 1603 was followed by several years of significant plague mortality: in Graunt's words, 'the *Plague* of 1603 lasted eight years'.[70] Perhaps significantly, this period saw a burgeoning literature of plague in English, as well as the first of Thomas Dekker's 'plague pamphlets'.[71] Careful study of the geography and chronology of plague deaths in these years could be very illuminating. Dekker's comment in 1606, that London was threatened by 'that Desolation, which now for three yeeres together hath houered round about thee', suggests that plague centred in the parishes outside the walls.[72] Statistics from weekly Bills provide some further clues, including the fact that plague deaths normally peaked in late September, but continued through the winter months, but for the most part research will need to focus on parish registers and changes in relative mortality.[73]

Plague was then (according to Graunt's tables) virtually absent from 1613 to 1624, but recurred in a major epidemic in 1625. However, Graunt notes that the number of those dying from other causes was also a huge increase over preceding years, leading him to conclude that 'there was errour in the Accompts . . . that is more died of the *Plague* then were accompted for under that name'.[74] If that is true of 1625, it might also lead us to query whether plague really was absent in the years preceding this epidemic, or whether there was reluctance or even wilful refusal to recognise it. The General Bill for 1624 records only eleven plague deaths, but the summer of that year saw multiple deaths attributed to spotted fever: John Chamberlain wrote that 318 died (of all causes) in one week in August 1624,

> a greater number than hath ben knowne these 15 or 16 yeares, and yet no mention of the plague. God kepe yt from among us . . . But this spotted feaver ys cousin german to yt [plague] at least, and makes as quicke riddance almost.

Two weeks later he noted that the weekly total had risen to 407, 'and yet we wil be acknowne of no infection'. Apart from infant deaths, 'most of the rest [were] carried away by this spotted feaver'.[75]

The authorities were apparently slow to acknowledge plague in 1625. Deaths were rising as early as April 1625, but 'the physicians do in a manner agree that this sicknes is not directly the plague, as not having any sore or any such like accident, but only contagious in a bloud or kindred'.[76] Attributed plague deaths, however, rose unevenly from April to June, and dramatically from late June, peaking in the third week of August. For the year as a whole, mortality for the city parishes and the outparishes in Middlesex and Surrey totalled 54,265, of which 35,417 were attributed to plague.[77] An additional Bill covering Westminster, Lambeth, Newington, Islington, Hackney, and Stepney adds 8,736 deaths, including 5,896 of plague, making the total 63,001, with 41,313 of plague.[78] No report of all causes seems to survive, to support or counter Graunt's comment that many plague deaths went unreported. Cummins, Kelly and Ó Gráda note that the Bills' figures for 1625 (total mortality) are higher than those they calculated from parish registers, implying that in some cases parish registration failed to keep pace with the epidemic.[79]

1627, 1628, and 1629 were virtually free from plague, according to Graunt's tables.[80] The pattern changed again in the 1630s, with no sharp dichotomy between major plague years and years of virtual absence. 1630 saw a comparatively mild outbreak, with 1,317 plague deaths, running over into the next year (274 plague deaths).[81] Nevertheless, Plague Orders were issued and Bartholomew Fair prohibited, and 1630 was noted as a plague year in a number of contemporary composite plague Bills, published during one epidemic, but listing deaths in previous plague years.[82] Most of the plague deaths in 1630 were in the suburbs, particularly to the east: St. Botolph Aldgate suffered 168 deaths, St. Mary Whitechapel 226.[83] 1636 was a more serious epidemic, if not on the scale of 1625, with 27,415 deaths, including 12,102 of plague, and was followed by 3,603 plague deaths in 1637. The year 1636 tends to be neglected in the study of major plague years, but the disease was widespread (only twelve parishes reported no plague deaths) and in some areas quite severe, with two clusters of infection within the walls around Aldersgate and Old Fish Street.[84] The epidemic appears to have started comparatively late, with no sharp rise in plague deaths until the end of July, but it persisted: though the peak number of deaths, 928, occurred in the week ending 29 September, there was a late upsurge to 838 deaths as late as 3 November.[85] In 1625, by comparison, all parishes but one were infected at some time, and the highest weekly mortality, 4,463, fell in mid-August.[86]

As Graunt noted, the plague of 1636 was followed by over a decade in which in most years 'there died [of plague] 2000 *per annum* one with another, and never under 300'.[87] The 1640s included nine years of minor to medium plague incidence, rising to a peak of 3,597 plague deaths in 1647. In all, some 15,000 people died of plague between 1640 and 1648.[88] Though spread out over time, this is a significant total; Londoners must have been very conscious of the lurking presence of the disease, 'this heavie and contagious time of the plague in London',[89] among all the other troubles besetting them. Fasting and public prayers to avert the plague were ordered in July 1640.[90] Plague Orders were issued for London in 1641, 1644, and 1646, and a handful of spiritual and medical remedies were published.[91]

An array of sources is available to track the patterns of deaths and plague deaths in the 1630s and 1640s. Apart from the total mortality figures in Graunt, some of the composite Bills give weekly mortality totals for 1636 and 1637.[92] Original weekly Bills survive, somewhat sporadically but in some years in significant numbers, especially for 1642 and 1647.[93] Parish registers survive from *c.* 1640 for about ninety of the city's 116 parishes, and for several of the outparishes.[94] Graunt, who had access to yearly Bills no longer extant, compiled a table of 'Diseases and casualties' for the city and outparishes for 1629–1636 and 1647–1660, allowing mortality from other diseases to be compared with plague mortality in 1636 and 1647, as well as providing a broader picture of the diseases and complaints prevalent in non-plague years.[95]

In addition, there are possibilities for correlation of mortality data for this period with contemporary social and economic data. In 1631 the Mayor and Aldermen estimated the population of the city's twenty-six wards (a slightly smaller area than the 113 city parishes covered in the 'City and Liberties' of the Bills of Mortality) at 130,178, a figure that should probably be inflated by 5–10 per cent for the floating population.[96] Estimates of the numbers of communicants in each parish also survive for the mid-1630s, though they are more problematic.[97] The reassessment of rent values in the city-wide tithe survey of 1638 numbers tithe-paying households in most parishes and provides a basis for characterising parishes as more or less wealthy, and for identifying other important features such as the presence of numerous low-rent dwellings, alleys, and tenements.[98] A survey of divided houses in 1637 provides complementary information on living conditions, particularly in poorer areas where subdivision and inmating were common.[99] A study of this period of low-level but not insignificant plague mortality, set alongside Champion's work on the major epidemic of 1665, and using as wide a range of sources as possible, could significantly advance our understanding of the disease and its impact.

Plague mortality seems to have tailed off sharply after 1648. Graunt notes 611 plague deaths in 1648, sixty-seven in 1649, and fifteen in 1650. From 1650 to 1664, a total of 204 deaths were attributed to plague, with a high of thirty-six in 1659 but with annual deaths in single figures in some years.[100] Copies of Yearly Bills from 1657 to 1664 show deaths from plague occurring almost at random, but mostly in the inner suburbs: Cripplegate, Bishopsgate, Aldgate, Whitechapel, and Southwark.[101] The epidemic of 1665, therefore, struck a city that had been largely free from plague for nearly two decades, and which had not seen a major epidemic for forty years.

Eyewitness accounts and rich contemporary documentation for the 1665 plague have encouraged extensive study, notably by W. G. Bell in 1924, and more recently by Justin Champion and by Lloyd and Dorothy Moote; Cummins, Kelly, and Ó Gráda have added further insights.[102] The epidemic killed the largest number of any since the fourteenth-century Black Death (68,596 attributed plague deaths of 97,306 in all), though it may be that, in relation to London's size at the time, it was not worse than those of 1563, 1603, or 1625. It displayed the classic seasonality of a May–June inception, September peak, and autumn decline. It began in the northwest suburbs and spread unevenly across the metropolis. Twenty parishes were reporting plague deaths by the end of June, seventy-three by the end of July, and 118 by the end of August. Only one parish was spared, the tiny St. John the Evangelist, 0.8 acre (0.32 ha) in extent and with only twenty-two taxpaying households in 1638. In general, the inner suburban parishes were the worst affected, with mortality up to seven times normal, but more distant parishes within the Bills also saw high plague mortality, in part no doubt the result of the flight of Londoners from the city itself.[103]

The 1665 epidemic had abated significantly by November, though aftershocks continued through 1666: some 2,000 plague deaths were recorded in 1666, half of them in the outer suburban parishes. The Fire of September 1666 displaced a large population, mostly from within the walls, and disrupted record-keeping, but even allowing for this, plague – or deaths attributed to it – seems to have largely disappeared by 1668. Only thirty-five plague deaths were reported in 1668, two-thirds of them south of the river, and over the next decade, they dwindled to zero. The last two deaths attributed to plague were in Rotherhithe, in 1679. The Bills kept a column for plague deaths until 1700, but then silently omitted it.[104]

The long-term chronology of plague incidence in London thus comprises a number of features: major epidemic peaks in single isolated years with tens of thousands of deaths, years when plague was virtually absent, and several periods in which plague was widespread and a serious killer for a number of years at a time. As already suggested, careful study of these last should add valuable information on social and spatial incidence, patterns of transmission, and lethality.

## Seasonal patterns and coincident diseases

The strong seasonality of London plague epidemics, with early-summer onset, September peak, and virtual disappearance by December, has been widely observed and is important in two ways. Atypical plague seasonality appears to have mitigated severity in epidemic years: it seems that 1636, a 'minor' plague year, saw a late start to the plague season, with deaths still high in November, just before the (presumed) onset of colder weather – though even at its worst, the plague of 1636 killed many fewer than that of 1625, despite the continuing growth of the metropolis. Furthermore, seasonal variations in mortality can be used to identify epidemics of diseases other than plague, even when specific causes are not given, and to suggest more complex mixed epidemics than the Bills' insistence on plague implies. Graham Twigg analysed the timing of mortality in a number of epidemic years, identifying not only a plague-type mortality pattern (common also to other diseases), but also an enteric type and an extended type, and argued that other disease organisms surely played a part in overall mortality.[105] The persistence of typical plague seasonality of mortality in the late seventeenth century, especially in outer parishes, has been noted by Cummins, Kelly, and Ó Gráda as complicating the view that 'plague' had disappeared after 1670.[106]

Somewhere between seasonality and long-term chronology are the cyclical patterns of infectious diseases other than plague. The other 'epidemicall' diseases prevalent in London ('Purples, Spotted-Feaver, Small-Pox, and Measles', according to Graunt) had different cycles and recurrences, at times coinciding with plague. Unlike plague, however, these diseases killed significant numbers in most years, with regular peaks, suggesting they were both endemic and epidemic.[107] Smallpox was present in mid-seventeenth-century London and seems to have established itself as both endemic and epidemic by the 1650s, with a three- to four-year cycle. The category 'ague and fever', probably comprising both influenza and malaria, was a major killer, causing around 13.5 per cent of non-plague deaths over most of the seventeenth century. Severity varied over a five- or six-year cycle, from 9 or 10 per cent of deaths to 17–18 per cent in individual years. Typhus (purples and spotted fever) was similarly variable, but – assuming it has been correctly diagnosed – much less destructive, averaging 1 per cent of non-plague deaths.[108]

As Champion pointed out, deaths from several other causes peaked in 1665: analysis of the 'residue deaths' indicates a huge increase in spotted fever and fever, a notable increase in 'surfeit', and increases in childbed and infantile deaths. Even if some of the 'fever' deaths were misdiagnosed or concealed plague deaths, he says 'it seems likely that there were minor epidemics of other diseases'.[109] The physician Thomas Sydenham believed that the 1665 plague was preceded and accompanied by a similar but distinct pestilential fever, 'truly of the same Species with the Plague, only 'tis a degree below it'.[110] The pattern of rising mortality from other causes can be found in earlier epidemic years, including 1636 and 1624–1625.[111] It may be worth correlating the cycles of other diseases with plague years. And while deaths by cause are only available in the Bills in figures aggregated across the metropolis, and year-to-year instability is itself a characteristic of the mortality of the period, it may also be feasible to use the Bills to identify years with high mortality from a particular disease (such as smallpox in 1652, or fever in 1686) and then to seek to pinpoint this unusual mortality at a more local level.

## Localities and environments

Seasonality and geography intersect in the spread of plague in epidemic years: there was almost always an initial focus, from which plague both 'diffused' into contiguous parishes and jumped into more distant ones. Cummins, Kelly, and Ó Gráda note that major plagues before 1665 consistently began in parishes to the north and northwest of the city, especially St. Giles Cripplegate; in 1665 it began first in St. Giles in the Fields, further west.[112] Also important is the pattern of decline. Though the number of 'infected' parishes (reporting one or more plague deaths) built slowly as an epidemic developed, the disease lingered in a large number of parishes as total mortality declined. In 1665, the 267 plague dead in the week ending 20 June came from twenty parishes; the 281 dead in the week ending 19 December were scattered across sixty-eight parishes.[113]

The social topography and environmental character of early modern London have been discussed by a number of authors. Clearly, there was variation from place to place and over time, as London's population expanded from perhaps 60,000–80,000 in the mid-sixteenth century to over 400,000 by the 1660s. The greatest population growth was in the inner suburbs, also the site of high plague mortality rates from c. 1600; changing patterns of plague incidence must be set against a changing environmental background.[114] Overall environmental quality did decline over time, from the early sixteenth century onwards: occupational density increased generally, but especially in the inner suburbs, development spread ever wider, and there was less urban open space and less access to rural space. Greater problems of water supply and waste disposal were only partly met by civic regulation and private-public enterprises such as the New River.[115] There was undoubtedly more air pollution as the burning of seacoal increased, both domestically and in industrial processes.[116]

The general character of London's built environment is fairly easily summarised. Its physical form was complex, with buildings continuous and contiguous, and with many interconnections and intermixtures between inhabited units. While there was much new building in the sixteenth and seventeenth centuries, older buildings survived and were altered and adapted to new patterns of use and occupation. Houses were still largely timber-framed, filled and faced in brick and plaster, and with brick chimneys; most had tiled roofs. Some had brick-lined or stone cellars. Yards and gardens were valued amenities, but liable to be sacrificed when the demand for accommodation was high.[117]

The effects of early modern London's rapid demographic growth varied from place to place. In the city centre and the fashionable areas of the West End, high demand for property entailed high rents and encouraged frequent rebuilding and increasing building heights; in the inner suburbs, there was increased density in low-rise occupation, by means of subdivision, conversion, and building closes and alleys of small dwellings on back plots and gardens; in the outer suburbs, green fields were built over with new, usually cheap, housing.[118] Overall, the houses of the better-off and middling sort may well have become more comfortable, better heated and insulated and better furnished. But the general population rise entailed a substantial increase in the numbers of poor and precariously-living, and in the geographical spread of areas of poor housing.

A broad overview of London's social topography can be gained from city-wide surveys and returns, such as the assessment of rental values, to revise tithe valuations (in the city only) in 1638, and the hearth taxes of the early 1660s, which contrast the greater wealth of the city centre with the poorer periphery immediately inside and outside the walls; some other measures, such as the geography of rate support and redistribution, reiterate the pattern.[119] The specification in the hearth tax legislation that nobody occupying a house with more than two hearths should be eligible for exemption on grounds of poverty implicitly linked dwelling size and poverty, and mapping exempt or non-paying dwellings is another useful measure of relative poverty.[120] It is certainly true that the poor lived among the rich, with many small houses and alleys between and behind more prestigious properties, even in central areas. However, historians' focus on mean or median rents and the proportion of 'substantial' householders tends to overlook these poorer neighbours. There was probably a real difference between these mixed areas and the uniformly poorer suburbs, to which many uses and activities potentially prejudicial to health – noisome and industrial processes – had been relegated.[121]

The hearth tax also contributes to more qualitative measures of housing poverty as, for example, in the implications of house size: single households occupying larger houses enjoyed more space per person, with rooms for separate functions. Cooking facilities and food storage were usually better provided for if there was a separate kitchen. While not all rooms in a house with several hearths were necessarily kept heated, there was more space for work as well as recreation. Privacy and autonomy were more easily available. Other important amenities – room height; the quality of materials and construction; repairs and maintenance, especially against water ingress;

adequate heating, water supply, and waste disposal – were all likely concomitants of larger and more expensive housing. It is worth noting, however – if it is argued that rats were a factor in the transmission of early modern plague – Twigg's observation that the black rat 'in modern times . . . has selected the well-to-do parts of the city where warmth was greater and food more plentiful', and might well have done the same in the sixteenth and seventeenth centuries.[122]

Environmental factors played a part in early modern views on plague, even if they were thought to operate in ways now unfamiliar to us. In modern times the association of dirt with germs and disease has been entangled in a circular argument about rats, fleas, and plague.[123] Early modern writers were certainly critical of accumulations of dirt and rubbish, poor street cleaning, and improper burial practices, but their concerns focused on the effect these had on air quality, a major factor in health, and on the possible contamination of water and foodstuffs.[124] 'An infected, corrupted and putrified Ayre' was identified as one of two 'especiall causes of the Pestilence' in 1603, and the *Certain necessary directions* of 1636 suggested that bonfires should be made in the streets 'for the correcting of the infectious aire'.[125] Simon Kellwaye in 1593 cited an array of environmental ills contributing to the spread of plague, including 'stincking doonghills, filthie and standing pooles of water, and unsavery smelles . . . neere the places where we dwell', but also noted climatic factors (both great heat and great rains) and unburied bodies after battles.[126] Similar themes persist through plague writings of the seventeenth century, sometimes with a more elaborately conceived epidemiology. Gideon Harvey in 1665 blamed 'nastiness of Kitchins, and . . . neglect of cleansing Gutters, sinks or Ditches, paving the Streets, burying the dead, removing Carrions and dead Carcases' as 'great occasions of Plague', because he believed that plague was generated within the earth, in which stinks and filth were 'coagulated into venene miasms'.[127] As already noted, the Plague Orders and proclamations required both public officers and private householders to 'take care for the due and orderly cleansing of the streets and priuate houses, which will auaile much in this case'.[128]

There was also a more general tendency to blame the living habits of the poor for their contribution to the disease.[129] John Stow's use of the term 'pestered' to denote overcrowding and alley-building in the suburbs is telling: St. Katherine's by the Tower was 'pestered with small tenements', Aldgate High Street 'pestered with diuers Allies'; 'From [Bethlem] Hospitall Northward vpon the stréetes side many houses haue beene built with alleyes backeward, of late time too much pestered with people (a great cause of infection) vp to the barres'.[130] The weekly *Intelligencer* for 14 August 1665 noted that plague was much increased 'in the Close and Filthy Allyes and Corners' about the city, but was hardly visible 'in the broad and open streets'; outside the city, it was concentrated in half a dozen outparishes, especially 'in the sluttish parts of those parishes where the poor are Crowded up together and in multitudes infect one another'.[131]

It is certainly clear that both respiratory and gastric diseases can be connected to housing defects and poor public hygiene – damp, cold, poor water supply, inadequate waste disposal – and when we can identify ailments by area, poorer areas seem to have higher death rates for such complaints, as for example the higher infant mortality in riverside parishes.[132] But this was not always a simple correlation: respiratory disease was high in crowded, suburban Aldgate in the early seventeenth century, but evidently less so in the poor but more open outer suburbs such as Stepney and Hackney.[133] In general, though, it is difficult to connect any infectious disease – including plague – directly to housing *per se* rather than to levels of poverty, overcrowding, nutrition, and lack of amenity. And even the correlation with poverty is uncertain. Champion documented a broadly concentric pattern of plague mortality across the whole metropolis in 1665, with the lowest rates in the centre and the highest rates towards the periphery, matching the general distribution of wealth. At the general level, he found a significant correlation between higher Crisis Mortality Ratios and areas where households averaged fewer hearths. However, analysing percentages of households infected and average deaths per infected household, he noted considerable local variation, suggesting that 'locational or spatial qualities' might be more strongly linked than social and economic categories.[134] And it should be noted that although plague mortality did get worse in the suburbs between the mid-sixteenth and the mid-seventeenth centuries, its relative impact was not greater in 1665 than in 1563, even though the metropolis was three times the size.[135]

## Conclusion: bubonic plague?

Finally, the perennial question of the identity of the disease that early modern Londoners, and their contemporaries elsewhere, called plague. Official publications, including the Bills of Mortality and the Plague Orders, envisaged a clear distinction between plague and other diseases, though some contemporary Londoners like Chamberlain seem to have been less confident, and others noted cases of misdiagnosis or misreporting.[136] While sixteenth- and seventeenth-century physicians and other writers described the disease they encountered and identified a number of direct and contributory causes in their pursuit of prevention and cure, confident diagnosis of a specific pathogen and mode of transmission was not made until the late nineteenth century. The identification of bubonic plague, *Pasteurella* (subsequently *Yersinia*) *pestis*, and the rat and rat-flea vectors as responsible for the Third Pandemic in east and south Asia seemed to solve the question of the Black Death and early modern European plagues and influenced almost a century of writing on the subject. As already noted, Graham Twigg challenged this diagnosis in 1984, and he and Samuel Cohn, in particular, have offered a detailed critique of the 'received wisdom' that the Second Plague Pandemic was (exclusively) bubonic plague, highlighting substantial inconsistencies between the characteristics and behaviours of the pre-modern and modern diseases, and difficulties with the rat-flea mode of transmission.[137] In Twigg's view, 'failure to acknowledge these [climatic] limitations on the part of plague has led to a tendency to adjust the biology of the disease and its vectors beyond their natural limits'.[138] Cohn has also demonstrated the entanglement of the evolving understanding of modern plague in the nineteenth and early twentieth centuries with ideas and assumptions about historic plagues.[139] A symposium on medieval plague at the Wellcome Trust Centre for the History of Medicine at University College London in 2006, bringing together experts from both sides of the argument, 'pinpointed very clearly where the difficulties lie in seeking to understand the causes and development of plague in Medieval Europe', but also usefully uncovered the thinking behind different approaches and conclusions.[140]

The question whether *Yersinia pestis* was involved in the early modern London plagues would seem to have been answered by the 2016 confirmation of traces of *Y. pestis* DNA in bodies excavated from an early modern pit burial, in a graveyard known to have received many plague victims between 1569 and 1665.[141] This discovery links with the identification of *Y. pestis* DNA in London burials from the Black Death of 1347–1351 to suggest continuity over the whole period.[142] However, this is by no means the end of the enquiry; while it answers one question, it leaves open many more. It does not necessarily help us to understand the impact and significance of the disease any better, and it remains the case that historic plague fails in many ways to conform to the epidemiology of modern bubonic plague. Some of these inconsistencies may be resolved by a less dogmatic presentation of the epidemiology of modern plague, including the exploration of alternative modes and agents of transmission – though there are difficulties with a simplistic assumption that the pneumonic variant resolves all problems – but it is vital that confirmation of the presence of *Y. pestis* does not foreclose critical questioning of the extent of its responsibility for all the deaths in epidemics classed as plague or lead to (renewed) attempts to force the historical evidence to fit given epidemiological models.[143] While further scientific research may be able to determine how the plague bacillus that has been identified in seventeenth-century London burials is related to other archaeologically-recovered strains of *Y. pestis*, and whether it had lethal capacity, for the historian it remains important to study and collate the documentary evidence, as free from epidemiological preconception as possible. Human actions may prove to be the key to variations in incidence and mortality, but those actions, and those variations, need to be carefully traced; 'we do know that we need to search out those connections'.[144]

## Notes

1   I thank John Henderson and Christos Lynteris for their helpful comments and insights – and their patience; also Kristin Heitman.
2   Creighton, *Epidemics*; Slack, *Plague*; Slack, *Impact*, Chapter 6; Sloane, *Black Death in London*.
3   The total number of deaths could have been c. 1.1–1.2 million. Cummins, Kelly, and Ó Gráda estimate that their database of 930,000 burial records 'comprises the individual burial records of over 80 per cent of those who died in London in this period': 'Living Standards', 3.
4   1,998 plague deaths were reported in 1666, 35 in 1667, fourteen in 1668, and thirty-four between 1669 and 1679: *A Collection*.

5 Bell, *Great Plague*; Champion, *London's Dreaded Visitation*; Porter, *Great Plague*; Moote and Moote, *Great Plague*; Wilson, *Plague in Shakespeare's London*; Slack, *Impact*; Twigg, *Bubonic Plague*. See also Porter, *Plagues*; Sutherland, 'When Was the Great Plague?'.

6 Creighton, *Epidemics*; Shrewsbury, *Bubonic Plague*.

7 Sloane, *Black Death*; Green, 'Pandemic Disease in the Medieval World'.

8 This problem, and its historiography, are lucidly set out in Nutton's preface and Introduction to *Pestilential Complexities*, 1–16.

9 Shrewsbury, *Bubonic Plague*; Slack, *Impact*; Appleby, 'The Disappearance of Plague'; Slack, 'The Disappearance of Plague'; Benedictow, *Black Death*.

10 Wilson, *Plague in Shakespeare's London*, 1–2, 37–38; Mullett, *Bubonic Plague*.

11 Twigg, *Black Death*.

12 Cohn, *Black Death Transformed*; Champion, *London's Dreaded Visitation*; Moote and Moote, *Great Plague*. But *Cf.* Porter, *Great Plague*, 21–23.

13 Scott and Duncan, *Return of the Black Death*; Twigg, *Bubonic Plague*; Nutton, *Pestilential Complexities*, 12–13.

14 Greenberg, 'Plague'.

15 Wilson, *Plague in Shakespeare's London*, 54–55.

16 Graunt, *Natural and Political Observations*. See also Robertson, 'Reckoning with London'.

17 Robertson, 'Reckoning with London'.

18 Chamberlain, *Letters of John Chamberlain*, Vol. *I*, 209, Vol. *II*, 612, 622; Pepys, *Diary*, Vol. *6*, 1665. Using parish maps to display the incidence of plague is common to modern writers including Slack, *Impact*, Champion, *London's Dreaded Visitation*, Twigg, *Black Death* and *Bubonic Plague*, and Cummins *et al.*, 'Living Standards'.

19 Jenner, 'Plague on a Page'; Monteyne, *Printed Image*, 73–112. See also Gilman, *Plague Writing*, 109–117; Harding, 'Reading Plague'.

20 *Certain necessary directions* described the quarantining of the sick as being 'according to the custom of Italy'. I owe this reference to John Henderson.

21 Slack, 'Metropolitan Government in Crisis'; Mullett, *Bubonic Plague*; LMA, COL/CC/01/01/022, ff. 284v–286v (May 1583).

22 *Orders to be vsed*; *Orders thought meet*; *A proclamation*; *Orders conceived*.

23 E.g. *Whereas the infection*; *By reason of grieuous visitation*.

24 E.g. LMA, COL/CA/01/01/074, ff. 135v–155v. See Harding, *The Dead and the Living*, Chapter 3; Harding, 'Epidemic Burial', 53–64.

25 LMA, COL/CC/01/01/022, ff. 284v–286v.

26 *Orders conceived*. See Jenner, 'Plague on a Page', for the dissemination of this image.

27 Pepys, *Diary*, Vol. *6*, 7 June 1665.

28 *Cf.* Newman, 'Shutt up'.

29 *Orders conceived*. *Cf.* Dorey, 'Controlling corruption', 24–41.

30 *Certain necessary directions*.

31 *Ibid.*

32 *Directions*.

33 Harding, 'Epidemic Burial'.

34 Slack, *Impact*, 22–30; *Cf.* Wear, 'Fear, Anxiety and the Plague'.

35 *Cf.* Wilson, *Plague in Shakespeare's London*; Barroll, *Politics, Plague, and Shakespeare's Theatre*.

36 *Orders conceived*.

37 *Ibid.*

38 E.g. *A thankes-giuing*.

39 Slack, *Impact*, especially Chapter 6, 'Metropolitan Crises'.

40 *Ibid.*, 154–169.

41 Champion, *London's Dreaded Visitation*.

42 Cummins, Kelly, and Ó Gráda, 'Living Standards'.

43 Creighton, *History of Epidemics*, Vol. *1*; Shrewsbury, *Bubonic Plague*. For a modern review of the disease and its problems, see Green, 'Pandemic Disease in the Medieval World'.

44 Though Creighton, *History of Epidemics, Vol. 1*, Chapters 6–9, provides rich evidence from a wide range of sources. See also Dyer, 'The English Sweating Sickness of 1551'; Fisher, 'Influenza and Inflation'; Moore, 'Jack Fisher's "Flu"'.
45 Slack, *Impact*, 148.
46 *Ibid.*; Creighton, *History of Epidemics, Vol. 1*, Chapter 6; Cummins, Kelly, and Ó Gráda, 'Living Standards'.
47 London parish registers consulted via Ancestry.com, and the volumes edited and printed by the Harleian Society. *Cf.* Forbes, *Chronicle from Aldgate*, 125–126.
48 Stow, *A summarie of Englyshe chronicles*, ff. 243–244.
49 Folger Shakespeare Library MS X.d.24; F.L., 'The Plague in London, 1563'.
50 The Folger memorandum and the mortality figures for 1563 will be discussed in a forthcoming blogpost on Folgerpedia.
51 Sutherland, 'When Was the Great Plague?'.
52 Cummins, Kelly, and Ó Gráda, 'Living Standards', 4.
53 LMA, P69/GEO/A/002/MS04792
54 Stow, 'Historical Memoranda, 1561-3'; Creighton, *History of Epidemics, Vol. 1*, 337–341.
55 Cummins, Kelly, and Ó Gráda, 'Living Standards', 12, Figure 4.
56 Slack, *Impact*, 151; Creighton, *History of Epidemics, Vol. 1*, 341.
57 Creighton, *History of Epidemics, Vol. 1*, 342–344
58 *The Number of all those that hath died.*
59 E.g. *St Dionis Backchurch*, 197–198; *St Peter Cornhill*, 129; *St Michael Cornhill*, 197–199.
60 E.g. *St Olave Hart Street*, 117–119,
61 Stow, *Annales*, 1274; Graunt, *Natural and Political Observations; Reflections on the Weekly Bills of Mortality; A Collection*; Bell, *London's Remembrancer*. Popular broadsides purporting to compare different plague years perpetuate confusion between 1592 and 1593: e.g. *Londons Lord have mercy upon us*. Berry, 'A London Plague Bill for 1592' explores the conflicting figures for 1592.
62 Cummins, Kelly, and Ó Gráda, 'Living Standards', 17, Figure 7.
63 Figures from *St. Martin in the Fields*, 131–139; Forbes, *Chronicle from Aldgate*, 59–61, 127.
64 Wilson notes 86 plague deaths reported between 1597 and 1600: *Plague in Shakespeare's London*, 85.
65 Wilson, *Plague in Shakespeare's London*, 86–93.
66 Chamberlain, *Letters of John Chamberlain, Vol. I*, 194.
67 Wilson, *Plague in Shakespeare's London*, 93–95.
68 Slack, *Impact*, 155, Figure 6.5.
69 *A True bill; A Collection.*
70 Graunt, *Natural and Political Observations*, 36.
71 Slack, 'Mirrors of health'; Wilson, *Plague Pamphlets of Thomas Dekker*.
72 Dekker, *The seuen deadly sinnes*, Introduction.
73 Wilson, *Plague in Shakespeare's London*, 186–187; *The true copie* (1603–1604); *The true copie* (1604); Bill of mortality.
74 Graunt, *Natural and Political Observations*, 35.
75 Chamberlain, *Letters of John Chamberlain, Vol. 2*, 576, 579.
76 *Ibid.*, 612.
77 *A Collection.*
78 *A generall or great bill.*
79 Cummins, Kelly, and Ó Gráda, 'Living Standards'.
80 Graunt, *Natural and Political Observations*, 75–76.
81 *Ibid.*
82 *Certaine statutes; A Proclamation; Cf. Lord have mercy upon us.*
83 *A Generall bill.*
84 Newman, 'Shutt up', examines the 1636 plague in the parish of St. Martin in the Fields; Figures from *The Mourning-cross.*
85 *Ibid.*
86 *A Collection.*

87  Graunt, *Natural and Political Observations*, 36.
88  *Ibid.*, 75–76.
89  *The stage-players complaint.*
90  *A forme of common prayer.*
91  Early English Books Online.
92  E.g. *The mourning-cross.*
93  Bodleian Library, Gough Add. MSS. I owe this reference to Paul Laxton.
94  *City of London Parish Registers: A Handlist.*
95  Graunt, *Natural and Political Observations. Cf.* Harding, 'Housing and Health'.
96  Harding, 'The Population of London'.
97  Tai Liu, *Puritan London.*
98  Dale, *The Inhabitants of London in 1638*; Jones, 'London in the Early Seventeenth Century'; Finlay, *Population and Metropolis*, 70–82, 168–172.
99  *Calendar of State Papers Domestic, 1637*, 178–183; The National Archives, London, SP16/359.
100  Graunt, *Natural and Political Observations.*
101  *A Collection.*
102  Bell, *The Great Plague*; Champion, *London's Dreaded Visitation*; Moote and Moote, *Great Plague*; Cummins, Kelly, and Ó Gráda, 'Living Standards'.
103  Figures from *London's Dreadful Visitation*. For localised impact, compare Slack, *Impact*, 154–156, Figures 6.3–6.6; Champion, *London's Dreaded Visitation*, 46–51, Figures. 17–22; Cummins, Kelly, and Ó Gráda, 'Living Standards', 18–21, Figure 8. For the epidemic's impact on places up to 25 miles from London, see Shrewsbury, *Bubonic Plague*, 481, Table 41.
104  *A Collection.*
105  Twigg, 'Plague in London'.
106  Cummins, Kelly, and Ó Gráda, 'Living Standards'.
107  Graunt, *Natural and Political Observations.*
108  Calculated from data in *A Collection.* The difficulty of distinguishing typhus from plague is noted by Cummins, Kelly, and Ó Gráda, 'Living Standards', 25, 31–32.
109  Champion, *London's Dreaded Visitation*, 27.
110  Pechey, *Collections of Acute Diseases*, 1–4.
111  Graunt, *Natural and Political Observations*; Chamberlain, *Letters of John Chamberlain, Vol. II*, 576, 578–579, 612.
112  Cummins, Kelly, and Ó Gráda, 'Living Standards', 18–19; *Cf.* Twigg, 'Plague in London', 5–7.
113  *A Collection* (1759).
114  Harding, 'The Population of London'; Slack, *Impact*, 154–156; Champion, *London's Dreaded Visitation*, 46–51, 101.
115  Brett-James, *The Growth of Stuart London.*
116  John Evelyn, *Fumifugium*, 5 and *passim*; Jenner, 'The Politics of London Air', 535–551. *Cf.* Cavert, 'The Environmental Policy of Charles I'; Cavert, *The Smoke of London.*
117  See Schofield, *Medieval London Houses*; Schofield, *The London Surveys of Ralph Treswell*; Harding, 'Families and Housing'; Gerhold, *London Planned.*
118  Power, 'East and West'; Power, 'The Social Topography of Restoration London'; Power, 'East London Housing'; Baer, 'Housing for the Lesser Sort'; Baer, 'Stuart London's Standard of Living'.
119  Dale, *Inhabitants of London in 1638*; Jones, 'London in the Early Seventeenth Century'; Finlay, *Population and Metropolis*, 70–82, 168–172; Wareham *et al.*, *London and Middlesex Hearth Tax Returns*; Power, 'The Social Topography of Restoration London'; Archer, *The Pursuit of Stability*, 151, Figure 1; Herlan, 'Social Articulation and the Configuration of Parochial Poverty'; *Cf.* Slack, *Impact.*
120  Wareham *et al.*, *London and Middlesex Hearth Tax Returns.*
121  Finlay, *Population and Metropolis*; Jones, 'London in the Early Seventeenth Century'.

122  Twigg, 'Plague in London', 15.
123  E.g. Creighton, *History of Epidemics, Vol. 1*, 173; Shrewsbury, *Bubonic Plague*, 227–228
124  Wear, 'Place, Health, and Disease'.
125  I.W., *A brief treatise of the plague; Certain necessary directions*, sig. c2.
126  Kellwaye, *A defensative against the plague*, f. 1v. These were among the factors cited by Galen: Slack, *Impact*, 27.
127  Harvey, *A Discourse of the Plague*, 5.
128  *Certain necessary directions.*
129  E.g. Slack, *Impact*, 27.
130  Stow, *Survay of London*, 89, 92, 128.
131  *The Intelligencer Published for the Satisfaction and Information of the People* (London), Issue 63, Monday 14 August 1665, 717. I owe this reference to Becky Wigley.
132  Finlay, *Population and Metropolis*, 101–106.
133  Harding, 'Housing and Health'.
134  Champion, *London's Dreaded Visitation*; *ibid.*, 'Epidemics and the Built Environment'.
135  Cummins, Kelly, and Ó Gráda, 'Living Standards'.
136  Chamberlain, *Letters of John Chamberlain*; Pepys, *Diary, Vol. 6*, 30–31 August 1665; Smyth, *Obituary*.
137  Twigg, *Black Death*; *ibid.*, *Bubonic Plague*, 15; Cohn, 'The Black Death'; *ibid.*, *The Black Death Transformed*. See also Champion, *London's Dreaded Visitation*, 6–10, 81–87.
138  Twigg, 'Plague in London', 1.
139  Cohn, *The Black Death Transformed*.
140  Nutton, *Pestilential Complexities*, vii.
141  Hartle, *The New Churchyard*; Harding, 'Epidemic Burial'.
142  Callaway, 'Plague Genome'.
143  *Cf.* 'Our results show that historical plague was caused by Y. pestis throughout Europe': Haensch *et al.*, 'Distinct Clones of Yersinia pestis Caused the Black Death'.
144  Green, 'Introduction', in: 'Pandemic Disease in the Medieval World'; Crespo and Lawrenz, 'Heterogeneous Immunological Landscapes and Medieval Plague'.

# References

## Manuscript sources

Folger Shakespeare Library, Washington, DC: MS X.d.24. 'The vicitacion of allmightie god wthin the cyttie of London', MS yearly bill of mortality for the calendar year 1563.
London Metropolitan Archives:
LMA, COL/CA/01/01/074: Corporation of London Repertory of the Court of Aldermen 70 (03 Nov. 1664–24 Oct. 1665), ff. 135v–155v.
LMA, COL/CC/01/01/022: Corporation of London, Journal of the Court of Common Council 21 (02 Nov. 1579–28 Oct. 1583).
LMA, P69/AND1/A/009: Burial register of St. Andrew by the Wardrobe, 1558–1850.
LMA, P69/GEO/A/002: Burial register of St. George Botolph Lane.
    The National Archives, London: TNA, SP16/359: Returns of divided houses, 1637.

## Early modern printed works

All bibliographical details and citations from early modern printed works are from Early English Books Online (eebo.chadwyck.com), last accessed April 2018.
[*Bill of mortality*] *from the [16 February] to the [23]* (London, 1608 [recte 1609]: STC (2nd ed.) 16743.4).

*A Collection of the Yearly Bills of Mortality from 1657 to 1758 inclusive* (London, printed for A. Millar in the Strand, 1759) (unpaginated).

*A forme of common prayer; to be used upon the eighth of July: on which day a fast is appointed by His Majesties proclamation, for the averting of the plague, and other judgements of God from this kingdom* (London, printed by Robert Barker, 1640: STC (2nd ed.) 16557).

*A generall bill for this present yeere, ending the 16 of December 1630* (London, printed by the Parish Clerks, 1630: STC (2nd ed.) 16743).

*A generall or great bill for this yeere of the whole number of burials, which haue beene buried of all diseases, and also of the plague in the citie of Westminster, Lambeth, Newington, Stepney, Hackney and Islington: from Thursday the 30. of December, 1624. to Thursday the 22. of December, 1625. According to the report made by the parish clarkes of the said parishes* (London, printed by William Stansby, 1625: STC (2nd ed.) 16741.7).

*A proclamation declaring His Maiesties pleasure touching orders to be obserued for preuention of dispersing the plague [By the King.]* (London, printed by Robert Barker, printer to the Kings most excellent Maiestie, 1636: STC (2nd ed.) 9063).

*A proclamation prohibiting the keeping of Bartholomew Fayre, Sturbridge Fayre, and Our Lady Fayre in Southwarke [By the King.]* (London, printed by Robert Barker, 1630: STC (2nd ed.) 8960).

*A thankes-giuing, for the decreasing and hope of the removing of the plague being a sermon preached at St. Pauls in London, vpon the 1. of Ianuary, 1636* [1637]. By Iohn Squier (London, printed by B. A[lsop] and T. F[awcet] for Iohn Clark, 1637: STC (2nd ed.) 23119).

*A True bill of the whole number that hath died in the cittie of London, . . . to this present month of October the sixt day, 1603* (London, printed by I.R. for Iohn Trundle, 1603: STC (2nd ed.) 16743.2).

Bell, John, *London's Remembrancer, or, A true accompt of every particular weeks christnings and mortality in all the years of pestilence . . . being xviii years* (London, printed by E. Cotes, 1665: Wing B1800).

*By reason of grieuous visitation in this time of the great contagion of the plague amongst our poore subiects [Charles by the grace of God, . . . ]* (London, printed by Robert Barker, 1636: STC (2nd ed.) 9074).

*Certain necessary directions, aswell for the cure of the plague as for preuenting the infection* (London, printed by Robert Barker, 1636: STC (2nd ed.) 16769.5)

*Certaine statutes especially selected, and commanded by his Maiestie to be carefully put in execution by all iustices . . . against the infection of the plague* (London, printed by Robert Barker and Iohn Bill, 1630: STC (2nd ed.) 9342).

Dekker, Thomas, *The seuen deadly sinnes of London drawne in seuen seuerall coaches, through the seuen seuerall gates of the citie bringing the plague with them* (London, printed by E[dward] A[llde and S. Stafford] for Nathaniel Butter, 1606: STC (2nd ed.) 6522).

*Directions for the prevention and cure of the plague Fitted for the poorer sort* (London, printed by J. Grismond, 1665: Wing (2nd ed., 1994) W1577).

Evelyn, John, *Fumifugium, or, The inconveniencie of the aer and smoak of London dissipated* (London, printed by W. Godbid for Gabriel Bedel, and Thomas Collins, 1661: Wing E3488).

Graunt, John, *Natural and Political Observations Mentioned in a following Index, and made upon the Bills of Mortality* (London, printed by Thomas Roycroft, 1662: Wing G1599A).

Harvey, Gideon, M. D., *A discourse of the plague containing the nature, causes, signs, and presages of the pestilence in general, together with the state of the present contagion . . .* (London, printed for Nath. Brooke, 1665: Wing H1062)

I. W., *A brief treatise of the plague wherein is shewed the naturall cause of the plague, preservation from infection, way to cure the infected* (London: Valentine Simms, 1603), STC (2nd ed.) 24905.7.

Kellwaye, Simon, *A defensative against the plague* (London: printed by John Windet, 1593), STC (2nd ed.) 14917).

*London's dreadful visitation, or, A collection of all the bills of mortality for this present year beginning the 20th of December, 1664, and ending the 19th of December following: as also the general or whole years bill: according to the report made to the King's Most Excellent Majesty by the Company of Parish-Clerks of London* (London, Printed and are to be sold by E. Cotes, 1665: Wing G1593A).

*Londons Lord have mercy upon us. A true relation of seven mod[ern] plagues or visitations in London* (London, printed for Francis Coles, Thomas Vere, and John Wright, 1665: Wing (CD-ROM, 1996) L2937).

*Lord have mercy upon us* (London, printed for Thomas Lambert, 1636: STC (2nd ed.) 19251.3)

*Orders conceived and published by the Lord Major and aldermen of the city of London, concerning the infection of the plague* (London, printed by James Flesher, 1665: Wing O397).

*Orders thought meet by His Maiestie, and his Priuie Councell, to be executed throughout the counties of this realme . . . infected with the plague* (London, printed by Iohn Bill, Printer to the Kings most Excellent Maiestie, 1625: STC (2nd ed.) 9245.2).

*Orders to be vsed in the time of the infection of the plague* (London, printed by Isaac Iaggard, Printer to the Honourable City of London, 1625: STC (2nd ed.) 16729.1).

Pechey, John, *Collections of acute diseases. The second and third part. The second part, contains all that the learn'd and experience'd Dr. Sydenham, has written of the pestilential fever, and dreadful plague at London in the years 1665, 1666* (London, printed by J. R., 1688: Wing P1020A).

*Reflections on the Weekly Bills of Mortality for the Cities of London and Westminster, and the places adjacent* (London, printed for Samuel Speed, 1665: Wing G1603). Sometimes attributed to Graunt, but probably erroneously.

Stow, John, 'Historical Memoranda of John Stowe: General, 1561–1563', in *Three Fifteenth-Century Chronicles with Historical Memoranda by John Stowe*, James Gairdner (ed.) (London, 1880).

Stow, John, *A summarie of Englyshe chronicles conteynyng the true accompt of yeres, wherein euery kyng of this realme of England began theyr reigne, howe long they reigned: and what notable thynges hath bene doone durynge theyr reygnes. Wyth also the names and yeares of all the baylyffes, custos, maiors, and sheriffes of the citie of London, sens the Conqueste, dyligentely collected by Iohn Stovv citisen of London, in the yere of our Lorde God 1565. Whervnto is added a table in the end, conteynyng all the principall matters of this booke. Perused and allowed accordyng to the Quenes maiesties iniunction.* (London, by/at Thomas Marsh's, 1565: STC (2nd ed.) 23319).

Stow, John, *A suruay of London Contayning the originall, antiquity, increase, moderne estate, and description of that citie, written in the yeare 1598. by Iohn Stow citizen of London. Also an apologie (or defence) against the opinion of some men, concerning that citie, the greatnesse thereof. With an appendix, containing in Latine, Libellum de situ & nobilitate Londini: written by William Fitzstephen, in the raigne of Henry the second* (London, printed by [John Windet for] Iohn Wolfe, printer to the honorable citie of London: and are to be sold at his shop within the Popes head Alley in Lombard street, 1598: STC (2nd ed.) 23341).

Stow, John, *The annales of England faithfully collected out of the most autenticall authors, records, and other monuments of antiquitie, lately corrected, encreased, and continued, from the first inhabitation vntill this present yeere 1600 By Iohn Stovv citizen of London* (London, printed for Ralfe Newbery, 1600: STC (2nd ed.) 23335, p. 1274).

*The Intelligencer Published for the Satisfaction and Information of the People* [BL, Burney Collection of Newspapers] (London, 1665).

*The Mourning-cross: or, England's Lord have mercy upon us* (London, printed by Tho. Milbourn, 1665: Wing (2nd ed.) M2991B).

*The number of all those that hath dyed in the Citie of London & the liberties of the same, from the 28, of December 1581. vnto the 27, of December 1582* (London, printed by J. Charlewood, after 1582): STC (2nd ed.) 16738.5).

*The stage-players complaint . . . In this heavie and contagious time of the plague in London* (London, printed for Tho: Bates, 1641: Wing (2nd ed.) S5162).

*The true copie of all the burials and christnings aswell within the city of London as the liberties thereof, as in other parishes in the skirts of the city and out of the freedome according to the report made to the Kings Most Excellent Maiestie / by the Company of Parish Clerkes of the said city . . .* [1 Sept. 1603-16 Feb. 1603/4 and 29 Dec. 1603 – 12 April 1604] (London, Printed by Iohn Windet, printer to the honourable city of London, 1603–1604: STC (2nd ed.) 16743.10).

*The true copie of all the burials and christnings aswell within the city of London as the liberties thereof, as in other parishes in the skirts of the city and out of the freedome, according to the report made to the Kings most excellent Maiestie by the Company of Parish Clearks of the said city . . .* [24 May 1604 to 21 June 1604] (London, Printed by Iohn Windet, printer to the honourable city of London, 1604: STC (2nd ed.) 16743.11).

*Whereas the infection of the plague is daily dispersed [By the Major.]* (London, printed by Isaac Iaggard, 1625: STC (2nd ed.) 16729.2).

## Secondary works

Appleby, Andrew, 'The Disappearance of Plague: A Continuing Puzzle', *Economic History Review*, 33 (1980), 161–173.

Archer, Ian W., *The Pursuit of Stability. Social Relations in Elizabethan London* (Cambridge, UK: Cambridge University Press, 1991).

Baer, William C., 'Housing for the Lesser Sort in Stuart London: Findings from Certificates and Returns of Divided Houses', *London Journal*, 33, 1 (2008), 61–88.

Baer, William C., 'Stuart London's Standard of Living: Re-examining the Settlement of Tithes of 1638 for Rents, Income, and Poverty', *Economic History Review*, 63, 3 (2010) 612–637.

Barroll, L., *Politics, Plague, and Shakespeare's Theatre: the Stuart Years* (Ithaca, NY: Cornell University Press, 1991).

Bell, Walter George, *The Great Plague in London in 1665* (London: John Lane The Bodley Head Ltd., 1924).

Benedictow, Ole J., *The Black Death, 1346–1352: The Complete History* (Woodbridge: Boydell Press, 2004).

Berry, H., 'A London Plague Bill for 1592, Crich, and Goodwyffe Hurde', *English Literary Renaissance*, 25, 1 (1995), 3–25.

Brett-James, Norman G., *The Growth of Stuart London* (London: George Allen & Unwin Ltd., 1935).

*Calendar of State Papers Domestic, 1637* (London: Longmans, Green, Reader and Dyer, 1868).

Callaway, Ewen, 'Plague Genome: The Black Death Decoded', *Nature*, 478 (2011), 444–446.

Cavert, William M., 'The Environmental Policy of Charles I: Coal Smoke and the English Monarchy, 1624–1640', *Journal of British Studies*, 53, 2 (2014), 310–333

Cavert, William M., *The Smoke of London. Energy and Environment in the Early Modern City* (Cambridge, UK: Cambridge University Press, 2016).

Chamberlain, John, *The Letters of John Chamberlain*, N. E. McClure (ed.) (Philadelphia: American Philosophical Society, 1939)

Champion, Justin A. I. (ed.), *Epidemic Disease in London* (London: Centre for Metropolitan History, Institute of Historical Research, University of London, 1993).

Champion, Justin A. I., 'Epidemics and the Built Environment in 1665', in: Justin A. I. Champion (ed.), *Epidemic Disease in London* (London: Centre for Metropolitan History, Institute of Historical Research, University of London, 1993), 35–52.

Champion, Justin A. I., *London's Dreaded Visitation: The Social Geography of the Great Plague in 1665* (London: Historical Geography Research Group, 1995).

*City of London Parish Registers: A Handlist of Parish Registers, Register Transcripts and Related Records at Guildhall Library* (London: Guildhall Library Publications, seventh revised edition, 1999).

Cohn, Samuel K., 'The Black Death: End of a Paradigm', *American Historical Review*, 107 (2002), 703–738.

Cohn, Samuel K., *The Black Death Transformed: Disease and Culture in Early Renaissance Europe* (London: Arnold, 2002).

Creighton, Charles, *A History of Epidemics in Britain from A.D. 664 to the Extinction of the Plague, 2 Vols.* (Cambridge, 1891, 1894; second edition, with additional material by D. E. C. Eversley and others, London: Frank Cass & Co. Ltd., 1965. All references are to the second edition).

Crespo, Fabian and Matthew B. Lawrenz, 'Heterogeneous Immunological Landscapes and Medieval Plague: An Invitation to a New Dialogue between Historians and Immunologists', in: Monica H. Green, (ed.), 'Pandemic Disease in the Medieval World: Rethinking the Black Death', *The Medieval Globe*, 1 (2014), 229–258: http://scholarworks. wmich.edu/medieval_globe/1.

Cummins, Neil, Morgan Kelly, and Cormac Ó Gráda, 'Living Standards and Plague in London, 1560–1665', *Economic History Review*, 69 (2016), 3–34.

Dale, T. C. (ed.), *The Inhabitants of London in 1638, ed. from MS. 272 in Lambeth Palace Library* (London: Society of Genealogists, 1931).

Dorey, Margaret, 'Controlling Corruption: Regulating Meat Consumption as a Preventative to Plague in Seventeenth-Century London', *Urban History*, 36, 1 (2009), 24–41.

Dyer, Alan, 'The English Sweating Sickness of 1551: An Epidemic Anatomized', *Medical History*, 41 (1997), 362–384.

F. L., 'The Plague in London, 1563', *Notes and Queries*, II, VI, 1912, 384–385.

Finlay, Roger A. P., *Population and Metropolis: The Demography of London, 1580–1650* (Cambridge, UK: Cambridge University Press, 1981)

Fisher, F. J., 'Influenza and Inflation in Tudor England', *Economic History Review*, 18 (1965), 120–129.

Forbes, T. R., *Chronicle from Aldgate: London* (New Haven and London: Yale University Press, 1971)

Gerhold, Dorian, *London Planned* (London: London Topographical Society, 2016).

Gilman, Ernest B., *Plague Writing in Early Modern England* (Chicago and London: University of Chicago Press, 2009).

Green, Monica H., 'Introduction', in *ibid.* (ed.), 'Pandemic Disease in the Medieval World: Rethinking the Black Death', *The Medieval Globe*, 1 (2014), 9–26: http://scholarworks. wmich.edu/medieval_globe/1.

Green, Monica H. (ed.), 'Pandemic Disease in the Medieval World: Rethinking the Black Death', *The Medieval Globe*, 1 (2014): http://scholarworks.wmich.edu/medieval_ globe/1.

Greenberg, Stephen, 'Plague, the Printing Press, and Public Health in Seventeenth-Century London', *The Huntington Library Quarterly*, 67, 4 (2004), 508–527.

Haensch, Stephanie, Raffaella Bianucci, Michel Signoli, Minoarisoa Rajerison, Michael Schultz, Sacha Kacki, Marco Vermunt, Darlene A. Weston, Derek Hurst, Mark Achtman, Elisabeth Carniel, and Barbara Bramanti, 'Distinct Clones of Yersinia Pestis Caused the Black Death', *PLoS Pathog*, 6, 10, e1001134 (2010): https://doi.org/10.1371/journal.ppat.1001134.

Harding, Vanessa, 'The Population of London, 1550–1700: A Review of the Published Evidence', *London Journal*, 15 (1990), 111–128.

Harding, Vanessa, 'Epidemic Burial', in: Justin A. I. Champion (ed.), *Epidemic Disease in London* (London: Centre for Metropolitan History, Institute of Historical Research, University of London, 1993), 53–64.

Harding, Vanessa, 'Families and Housing in Seventeenth-Century London', *Parergon*, 24, 2 (2007), 115–138.

Harding, Vanessa, 'Housing and Health in Early Modern London', in: V. Berridge and M. Gorsky (eds.), *Environment, Health and History* (Basingstoke: Palgrave Macmillan, 2011).

Harding, Vanessa, 'Reading Plague in Early Modern London', *Social History of Medicine*, forthcoming 2018.

Harding, Vanessa, *The Dead and the Living in Paris and London, 1500–1670* (Cambridge, UK: Cambridge University Press, 2002).

Hartle, Robert, *The New Churchyard: From Moorfields Marsh to Bethlem Burial Ground, Brokers Row and Liverpool Street* (London: MOLA, Crossrail Archaeology Series 10, 2017).

Herlan, Ronald W., 'Social Articulation and the Configuration of Parochial Poverty in London on the Eve of the Restoration', *Guildhall Studies in London History*, 2 (1976), 43–53.

Jenner, Mark S. R., 'Plague on a Page: Lord Have Mercy Upon Us in Early Modern London', *Seventeenth Century*, 27, 3 (2012), 255–286.

Jenner, Mark S. R., 'The Politics of London Air: John Evelyn's *Fumifugium* and the Restoration', *Historical Journal*, 38, 3 (1995), 535–551.

Jones, Emrys, 'London in the Early Seventeenth Century: An Ecological Approach', *London Journal*, 6 (1980), 123–133.

Monteyne, Joseph, *The Printed Image in Early Modern London: Urban Space, Visual Representation, and Social Exchange* (Aldershot: Ashgate, 2007).

Moore, John S., 'Jack Fisher's "Flu: A Virus still Virulent"', *Economic History Review*, 47, (1994), 359–361.

Moote, A. Lloyd and Dorothy C., *The Great Plague: The Story of London's Most Deadly Year* (Baltimore: Johns Hopkins University Press, 2004).

Mullett, Charles F., *The Bubonic Plague in England. An Essay in the History of Preventive Medicine* (University of Kentucky Press: Lexington, 1956).

Newman, Kira L. S., '"Shut upp": Bubonic Plague and Quarantine in Early Modern England', *Journal of Social History*, 45, 3 (2012), 809–834.

Nutton, Vivian (ed.), 'Pestilential Complexities: Understanding Medieval Plague', *Medical History*, Supplement 27 (2008).

Pepys, Samuel, *Diary of Samuel Pepys, 11 Vols*, Robert Latham and W. Matthews (ed.). (London: Bell, 1970–1983).

Pepys, Samuel, *The Diary of Samuel Pepys, 1660–1669*, Robert Latham and W. Matthews (ed.) (London: HarperCollins Publishers, 2010).

Porter, Stephen, *The Great Plague* (Stroud: Sutton Publishing, 2000).

Porter, Stephen, *The Plagues of London* (Stroud: Tempus, 2008).

Power, Michael J., 'East and West in Early Modern London', in: E. W. Ives, R. J. Knecht, and J. J. Scarisbrick, (eds.), *Wealth and Power in Tudor England* (London: Athlone Press, 1978), 167–185.

Power, Michael J., 'East London Housing in the Seventeenth Century', in: Peter Clark and Paul Slack (eds.), *Crisis and Order in English Towns 1500–1700* (London: Routledge and Kegan Paul, 1972), 237–262.

Power, Michael J., 'The Social Topography of Restoration London', in: A. L. Beier and Roger Finlay (eds.), *London 1500–1700, the Making of the Metropolis* (London: Longman, 1986), 199–223.

Robertson, James C., 'Reckoning with London: Interpreting the Bills of Mortality before John Graunt', *Urban History*, 23 (1996), 325–350.

Schofield, John, *Medieval London Houses* (London: Yale University Press, 1995).

Schofield, John, *The London Surveys of Ralph Treswell* (London: London Topographical Society, 1987).

Scott, Susan and Christopher Duncan, *Return of the Black Death: The World's Greatest Serial Killer* (Chichester: Wiley, 2004).

Shrewsbury, J. F. D., *A History of Bubonic Plague in the British Isles* (Cambridge, UK: Cambridge University Press, 1971).

Slack, Paul, 'Metropolitan Government in Crisis: The Response to Plague', in: A. L. Beier and Roger Finlay (eds.), *London 1500–1700, the Making of the Metropolis* (London: Longman, 1986), 60–81.

Slack, Paul, 'Mirrors of Health and Treasures of Poor Men: The Uses of the Vernacular Medical Literature of Tudor England', in: C. Webster (ed.), *Health, Medicine and Mortality in the 16th Century* (Cambridge, UK: Cambridge University Press, 1979), 237–274.

Slack, Paul, 'The Disappearance of Plague: An Alternative View', *Economic History Review*, 34 (1981), 469–476.

Slack, Paul, *Plague: A Very Short History* (Oxford: Oxford University Press, 2012)

Slack, Paul, *The Impact of Plague on Tudor and Stuart England* (Oxford: Oxford University Press, 1985).

Sloane, Barney, *The Black Death in London* (Stroud: History, 2011).

St. Dionis Backchurch, *The Reiester Booke of Saynte De'nis, Backchurch Parishe (City of London) for Maryages, Christenyges, and Buryalles, Begynnynge in the Yeare of Our Lord God 1538*, Vol. 3, Joseph Lemuel Chester (ed.) (London: Harleian Society, Registers, 1878).

St. Dunstan East, *The Register of St. Dunstan in the East, London, Pt. 1, Vol. 69*, A.W. Hughes Clarke (trans. and ed.) (London: Harleian Society, Registers, 1939).

St. Martin in the Fields, *A Register of Baptisms, Marriages and Burials in the Parish of St. Martin in the Fields in the County of Middlesex from 1550 to* 1619, Vol. 25, Thomas Mason (ed.) (London: Harleian Society Registers, 1898).

St. Michael Cornhill, *The Parish Registers of St. Michael, Cornhill, London: Containing the Marriages, Baptisms, and Burials from 1546 to 1754, Vol. 7*, Joseph Lemuel Chester (ed.) (London: Harleian Society, Registers, 1882).

St. Olave Hart Street, *The Registers of St. Olave, Hart Street, London. 1563–1700, Vol. 46*, W. Bruce Bannerman (ed.) (London: Harleian Society, Registers, 1916).

St. Peter Cornhill, *A Register of all the Christninges, Burialles & Weddinges Within the Parish of Saint Peeters Upon Cornhill: Beginning at the Raigne of Our Most Soueraigne Ladie Queen Elizabeth, Vol. 1*, Granville W. G. Leveson Gower (ed.) (London: Harleian Society, Registers, 1877).

Sutherland, Ian, 'When Was the Great Plague? Mortality in London, 1563–1665', in: D. V. Glass and R. Revelle (eds.), *Population and Social Change* (London: Edward Arnold, 1972), 287–320.

Tai Liu, *Puritan London: A Study of Religion and Society in the City Parishes* (Newark, NJ: Princeton University Press, 1986).

Twigg, Graham, 'Plague in London: Spatial and Temporal Aspects of Mortality', in: Justin A. I. Champion (ed.), *Epidemic Disease in London* (London: Centre for Metropolitan History, Institute of Historical Research, University of London, 1993), 1–17.

Twigg, Graham, *Bubonic Plague: A Much Misunderstood Disease* (Ascot: Derwent Press, 2013).

Twigg, Graham, *The Black Death: A Biological Reappraisal* (London: Batsford, 1984).

Wareham, A., M. Davies, C. Ferguson, V. Harding, and E. Parkinson (eds.), *The London and Middlesex Hearth Tax Returns* (London: British Academy, 2014).

Wear, Andrew, 'Fear, Anxiety and the Plague in Early Modern England: Religious and Medical Responses', in J. R. Hinnells and Roy Porter (eds.), *Religion, Health and Suffering* (London and New York: Kegan Paul International, 1999), 339–363.

Wear, Andrew, 'Place, Health, and Disease: The Airs, Waters, Places Tradition in Early Modern England and North America', *Journal of Medieval and Early Modern Studies*, 38, 3 (2008), 443–465.

Wilson, F. P. (ed.), *The Plague Pamphlets of Thomas Dekker* (Oxford: Clarendon Press, 1925).

Wilson, F. P., *The Plague in Shakespeare's London* (Oxford: Oxford University Press, 1927).

# 3

# 'FILTH IS THE MOTHER OF CORRUPTION'[1]

## Plague, the poor, and the environment in early modern Florence

*John Henderson*

**11 August 1630, the Quarter of S. Ambrogio**

Between Via Nuova and [Borgo] Pinti in the courtyard of the house of Monna Caterina, widow of Jacopo the coachman, and Monna Piera di Zanobi: redo the straw mattresses because they smell, and it is necessary to burn the old ones because there is a great stink. There are seven people to a room and they do everything in the same courtyard; to the left in the room of Monna Dianora there is a fetid bed, which could create plague where it has not been up until now, thus burn and replace it.[2]

This passage from a sanitary survey of Florence reflects the concerns of contemporaries in seventeenth-century Tuscany about the physical environment and how the way that people lived influenced their health. The matter-of-fact description spells out the very cramped living conditions in one of the poorer parts of the city, with seven people sleeping in one room on filthy bedding and *paliasses* or straw mattresses. The real fear was that because these conditions created a great stink and fetid air, they would create plague; in fact, by mid-August 1630 their fears were realised when an epidemic broke out in the city. It is this theme of poverty, the physical environment, and plague, which is at the centre of this chapter. However, in order to properly understand the reason for this intense interest in the connection between the fabric of the city, disease, and the living conditions of the poor, we have to take a step back to place this survey and the epidemic of plague of 1630–1631 in Florence within a wider chronological, administrative, and above all medical context.

## The 'city is [like] a hospital': the tradition of sanitary legislation

A major theme of contemporary Florentine treatises written about the 'pestilential contagious diseases' of 1630–1631 was that the insanitary conditions associated with poverty and poor housing was one of the fundamental causes of plague.[3] This belief had a long and venerable tradition in late medieval medical treatises. It was, in particular, the poisonous vapours generated, in the words of an eminent contemporary physician Stefano Roderico De Castro, by 'earthquakes, unburied bodies, stagnant and fetid water', which caused plague.[4] Insanitary conditions were seen as particularly bad in cities through the effluence generated by humans living in close proximity. De Castro underlined why cities were so unhealthy:

> crowds of sick people and of those who care for them can besmirch the air, and the proof is clear; as one always flees the air inside hospitals, because the breath of the sick fills them with bad vapours. I imagine that similarly at a time when there are many sick people in a city, that city is [like] a hospital.[5]

The belief in the association between bad air and disease had also underlain sanitary legislation from well before the Black Death, when medieval states and cities had enacted measures to clean up the environment, from the disposal of human waste and the banning of the butchery of animals in city centres, as discussed by Carole Rawcliffe in Chapter 1 in this volume on butchery and plague in late medieval England. At the time of the Black Death, Giovanni Boccaccio recorded in his Introduction to *The Decameron*:

> in that [pestilence] no wisdom or measure was of any use, such as the clearing of the city of much refuse by officials appointed for that purpose, and the prohibition of any person from entering [the city] and many counsels [Consilia] given for the preservation of health.[6]

In Florence, as Boccaccio records, as in many cities and towns across Italy, magistrates had been established in order to investigate infractions of the sanitary legislation, whether deriving from reports of the officials themselves or of concerned citizens.[7] However, despite legislation and its enforcement, contemporaries complained stridently about high levels of stench, which convinced them that bad smells were the cause of plague. From the second half of the sixteenth century, these ideas became even better developed through the influence of the growing literature arguing for the close connection between the physical environment, health, and disease. disease. Particularly influential in this regard was the revival of Hippocrates' treatise *Airs, Waters and Places*. He emphasised the close connection between location and climate and hence the causative link between the health and disease of an area, whether urban or rural, and of local inhabitants.[8]

Even with this general awareness of the ever-increasing emphasis of the close association between insanitary conditions and disease, it is only relatively recently that historians have started to examine the impact of these ideas on government policy and the extent to which regulations were enforced.[9] This is a topic which has been studied more extensively for later periods through the emergence of the genre of medical topographies in the eighteenth century.[10] It has been argued for northern Italy that one impetus to a more general public awareness of the link between disease and the environment was the epidemic of plague of 1575. This was reflected in the explosion of broadsheets in Venice, Milan, and Bologna, giving instructions for citizens to keep the streets clean of refuse and excrement to prevent the spread of disease.[11]

Another important feature of government policy in the sixteenth century was the growing intolerance and fear of the poor, as they came increasingly to be seen as the source of infection.[12] This attitude was fuelled by the impact of the new epidemic of the Great Pox and exacerbated still further by the devastating plague epidemic of 1575–1576 in northern Italy.[13] Even so, reactions were tempered by the influence of the Counter-Reformation, which underlined the church's attitude towards the poor, who were also seen as worthy objects of redemption.[14] In Verona, for example, while the city expelled beggars, they also expressed pity for their plight. Carlo Borromeo, who gave his name to this epidemic, was famous for the help he gave to the poor, underlining the two sides of the motivation behind charity, compassion and fear.[15]

## The plague of 1630–1631

By the early seventeenth century, and in particular during the last epidemic to hit northern and central Italy between 1629 and 1633, the association between the physical environment and living conditions of the poor became even more entrenched and elaborated.[16] This chapter will concentrate on Florence, the capital of the Medicean Grand-Ducal state of Tuscany, where the epidemic started in August 1630 and lasted for about a year. Once plague had taken hold in the city, the period of worst mortality was in late autumn with a slow tailing off over the subsequent seven months. During the whole period in which plague was in the city, August 1630 to July 1631, about 12 per cent of the resident population of 75,000 had died.[17] This was a relatively low mortality rate when compared to cities further north, such as Milan and Venice, which suffered respectively from a 46 and 33 per cent mortality rate of populations in excess of 130,000, while some smaller centres were hit even more hard, such as Verona, which lost 57 per cent of its population.[18]

The fact that plague arrived in Tuscany almost two years after it had entered Italy, and six months after it had impacted on the cities in northern Italy, would have left the authorities with plenty of time to take precautionary measures to prevent its arrival, especially given the regular exchange of information concerning the threat and progress of epidemics between governments and health boards across the peninsula. The main strategies adopted to stop the plague from spreading into Tuscany included banning trade and commerce with infected states and then establishing *cordon sanitaires* around the frontiers of Tuscany.[19]

Once plague had broken out in the city, a separate set of controls was adopted, familiar from studies across renaissance and early modern Europe.[20] The city's Health Board, the Magistrato di Sanità, which we saw in genesis in Boccaccio's 'Introduction' to the *Decameron*, coordinated all operations not just outside, but also within the city: banning public assemblies, prohibiting the sale of cloth and clothes, quarantining the sick in their houses and in isolation hospitals or Lazaretti, and the burial of victims in special pits outside the city walls, all enforced by its own police officers and law courts.[21] Every resident was obliged to report the sick within their household or house, followed by the visit of the physician of the Sanità to ascertain if the ailment was an 'ordinary disease' or a 'contagious disease'. If anything suspicious was discovered, the patient was sent to the Lazaretto and members of the household were quarantined for twenty-two days either at home or in extramural isolation centres. The transportation of the sick and dead was performed by the Fraternity of the Misericordia. This was a brotherhood of voluntary laymen who dedicated themselves to charitable works and had been for over 140 years the main organisation in the city to man this emergency service during epidemics.[22] At the same time the clothes and bedding of the sick and dead were removed and taken to be burnt or aired for forty days, and the house was subsequently disinfected. A satirical view on these operations can be seen in a contemporary print of the Health Board operatives working in Rome during the 1656 plague, chucking out from a first floor the contents of an infected house for disinfection (see Figure 3.1).[23]

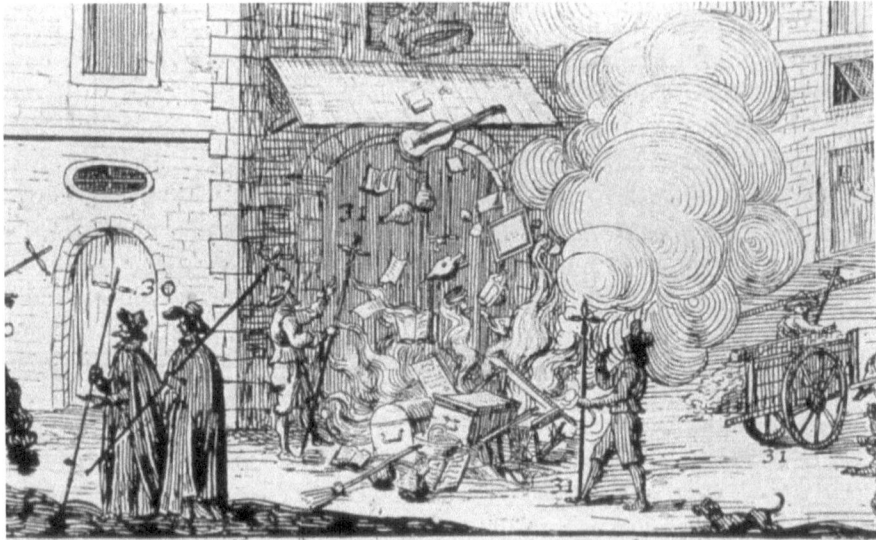

**FIGURE 3.1** 'Disinfection of goods from a plague house', *Scenes from the Plague in Rome of 1656* (credit: Wellcome Library, London)

All these measures were predicated on the belief that plague could be spread by individuals and materials, and in particular, cloth, which was seen as having the ability to hold within itself the 'seeds' of plague and hence the lengthy periods of disinfection through exposure to the air. Cloth had been at the centre of concerns of administrators and their medical advisers from the time of the Black Death onwards.[24]

## Medical theory: poverty, disease, and the environment

The increased emphasis in public health policy from the late sixteenth century on the relationship between poverty, disease, and the urban environment was discussed and explained in detail in a growing body of medical literature.[25] In addition to the influence of neo-Hippocratic ideas, contemporaries stressed the importance of the Galenic concept of the six non-naturals, those individual and environmental factors which influenced well-being.[26] The most crucial non-natural from our point of view was air, given that diseased air was seen as causing disease, and led, as we shall see, to the concentration by the authorities on insanitary conditions.[27] In Florence at the beginning of the epidemic in August 1630, the College of Physicians was asked by the Sanità to determine the nature of the disease, in order to provide the government with guidance over which prophylactic measures to adopt. This led in August to discussions and then debates being held at the highest medical and social levels. As the Librarian of the Grand Duke of Tuscany, Francesco Rondinelli, who wrote an official history of the epidemic, recorded:

> all the city was divided between [different] opinions: one that said it was a pest and these were called the Frightened Ones . . . The others said that they were ordinary sicknesses, which happened every year, caused by suffering and hardship.[28]

Although there was some disagreement about whether or not it was the 'contagious sickness', most medical experts did agree what caused the most immediate and readily observable effect of this epidemic, higher mortality among the poor. Rondinelli summarised briefly the most widely held medical explanation. He recorded that recently the poor had suffered considerably from a series of severe dearths when they had been forced to consume food and drink of poor quality. Indeed the 1620s had seen a series of famines and the subsequent outbreak of epidemics of typhus.[29] The dearths had led, according to some doctors, to the generation in the bodies of the poor of 'a great mass of bad humours', which had led to the creation in them of an 'extraordinary putrefaction, which even from a long distance and even for any occasion has become the pest'.[30]

Rondinelli reported here the ideas enunciated by two eminent physicians, Alessandro Righi and Stefano De Castro, who both advised the Sanità and then wrote treatises on plague.[31] Righi took the standard Galenic line and emphasised that not eating well increased the level of bad humours within the bodies of the poor and weakened their resistance to disease.[32] Stefano de Castro also argued that their wilful ignorance made them susceptible to disease. He portrayed the poor as refusing to believe it was necessary to keep clear of an infected person, who, although he might not have an evident '*segno del male*', could still be carrying the 'secret seed of contagion'.[33] Furthermore, he suggested, that the shortage of money of the poor meant they could not take the proper preventive measures against plague, such as buying aromatic herbs and spices to burn and perfume the air, all compounded by not having enough space to avoid mixing with infected people.[34]

If De Castro portrayed the poor as victims of their own prejudices and ignorance, Righi instead had a more fatalistic approach. According to him, it was in the very nature of the poor to attract disease, as he demonstrated by taking the Platonic analogy between the human body and the city. He likened the noble and robust organs, such as the heart, to the upper levels of society and the poor to the less noble and robust organs (veins, arteries, skin, and glands). The rich were seen as having the ability to expel unnecessary dangerous substances towards the outside and the lower organs. The poor, who did not possess the same ability, became the deposit of poisons: 'therefore . . . if the disease is in the city, they [the poor] receive it and retain it, as if they were the glands of society'.[35] This vision of society as a body was not just confined to the medical world. In Rome during the 1656 epidemic the Jesuit Sforza Pallavicino recorded that when plague had begun to spread through Trastevere a decision was made to place the poor sick into a Lazaretto in order to 'cut off, according to the rules of surgery, all that part that was weak and ignoble from the best parts of the body'.[36]

## Public health and preventive measures

Thus in Florence, as in Rome and elsewhere, medical men provided a justification for the measures taken by the Sanità to cope with the unfolding crisis of the plague epidemic. An important element of this was how they dealt with the poorer elements of society. Those at the very base of the social pile, beggars, were, as in other parts of Europe, divided between 'foreigners' and the locals; the former were expelled from the city, while the latter were sent to the Spedale dei Mendicanti, a special beggars' hostel in the parish of San Frediano, a working-class area south of the river.[37] As Rondinelli records, it was feared that beggars 'could catch the fire of the contagion and sow it through the city' in their search for alms.[38]

This association between poverty, insanitary housing, and the genesis and spread of plague was to have a long history, as reflected in studies of the Third Pandemic. This is a theme emphasised in Chapter 6 in this volume by Engelmann and Evans on late nineteenth and early twentieth-century America and India. Indeed the Board of Health in Honolulu argued in December 1899 that plague germs 'flourish in filth, in garbage and in damp, dark or foul places' (see Engelmann below). But there is another theme which the Second and Third Pandemics shared, the strong culture of blame; in Florence: beggars, the poor, prostitutes, and the Jews, compared with the Chinese population, whether in Honolulu, Hong Kong, or San Francisco (see also Peckham below).

The emphasis throughout Rondinelli's account reflected the prejudices and general attitudes towards the poor as the initiators of the epidemic and the cause of its spread. This was proved to the satisfaction of contemporaries because the highest mortality was recorded in the poorer areas of the city with high-density housing where households were crowded together. The first deaths were in three streets in the medieval centre (Via del Garbo, Canto alla Briga, and S. Pancrazio), from where it spread outwards to the rest of the city (see Figure 3.2).[39]

In each case the Sanità traced the cause of the infection to specific people, a cloth-merchant named Sisto Amici had had contact with the source of the infection in Trespiano, a village five miles to the north of the city; the wife of a man called 'Il Rovinato' ('the wreck'), who had looked after her sick sister and taken away a favourite shirt and given it to her daughter who promptly died; and the wife of the

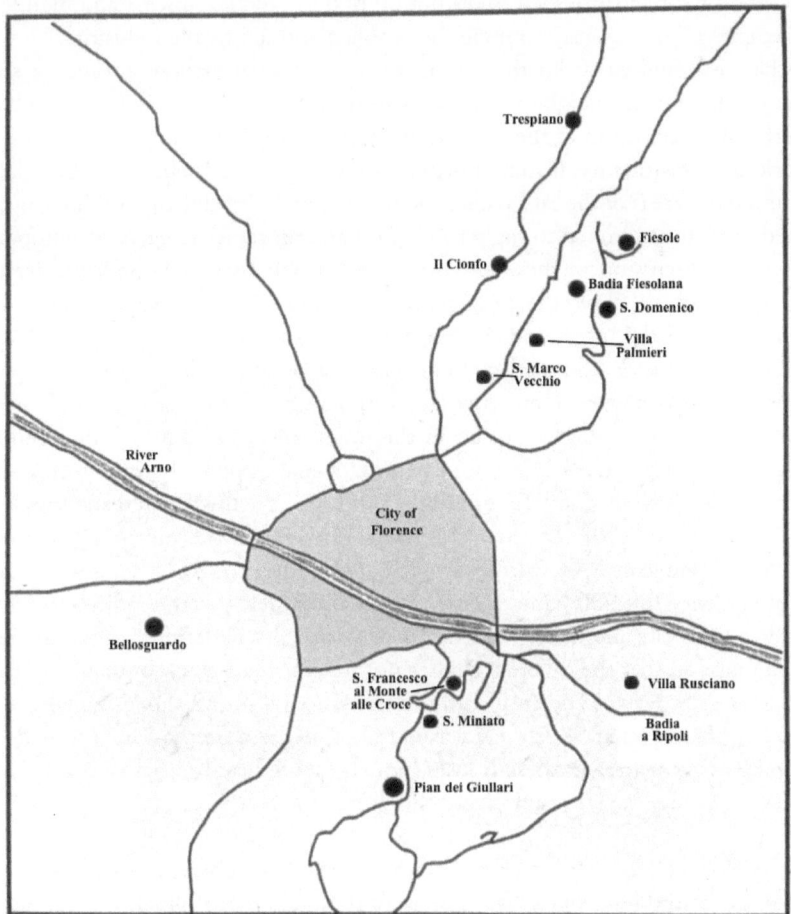

**FIGURE 3.2**  City of Florence with location of the first cases of plague, August 1630.
   Drawn by the author

baker Maestro Francesco at S. Pancrazio, who had nursed her dying daughter and had brought the disease back to her house, probably causing its further spread in the neighbourhood as the bakery would have been a hub of social activity.[40] All these individuals were portrayed by contemporary commentators as ignorant and irresponsible and having put their interests before that of the city. Evidence which appears to substantiate this claim can be found in the prosecutions of over 550 individuals for breaking the decrees and laws of the Sanità over the course of the epidemic. However, while the official version of events written by men like Rondinelli represents the opposition of authority and the poorer sorts, many cases reveal a more nuanced picture. Even if it is true there was deliberate criminal activity, such as the theft of goods from empty houses, judges were often lenient in their sentencing, recognising that much of the time these cases derived from the poorer sorts attempting to adopt a wide range of strategies to survive in an economically depressed environment, as plague regulations led to disruption of trade and commerce and high levels of unemployment, especially among the woollen and silk textile industries.[41]

What also emerges from these trial records is the surprising amount of social activity at family and neighbourhood levels during the plague.[42] This, combined with the close attention of the authorities to the living conditions of the poor, led to various levels of surveillance, not just to control social behaviour, but also to determine the areas of the city where the most crowded and insanitary housing was located, which was linked to higher infection and mortality rates. A contemporary anonymous discussion of these environmental problems emphasised two features of housing, which made the poor particularly susceptible to plague, particularly for those who lived in ground-floor apartments: a humid atmosphere, where the 'walls run with water' and the lack of proper ventilation.[43] All this was made worse because conditions were often crowded, with families of four or five children, and 'they do not have ventilation or air in the house and have only a little window'. Their poverty also meant they often had no 'benches or bed and hardly a straw mattress or a mattress of tow [hemp fibre]', and when beds were remade they were found to be mildewed, and their clothes were damp in the morning when they woke up. Conditions were further exacerbated during the forty-day total quarantine of Florence from 20 January 1631, when all residents were required to remain in their houses day and night, 'so living like this they will definitely die'. Indeed it was emphasised that they were a danger not just to themselves, but also to others: 'because if they get sick they infect the others who live above them'. Finally, it was rumoured that another health risk was in the offing because the Sanità intended to distribute coal for fires in these houses, which would lead to a 'great fear of some sickness', because 'coal would create the greatest damage [to health] because it is too hot'.[44]

It is probable that this document was written in February 1631 during the quarantine of the city, but it was precisely these concerns which lay behind the sanitary surveys of the poorest zones of the city six months earlier in August 1630, when a series of measures had been instituted to repair the systems for dealing with human waste, to replace mattresses and *paliasses* as well as to provide subsidies to the very poor. This grew out of an existing tradition of surveying insanitary conditions in Tuscany from the late sixteenth century, partly in response to epidemics of typhus, and in turn built on the surveying systems of the long tradition of tax and population censuses.[45] Such surveys also became more standard features of anti-plague measures plague in early modern Italy, as revealed by studies of Bologna in 1630 and Rome in 1656.[46]

## The sanitary survey in Florence, August to September 1630

The recognition of the close relationship between environment and plague in 1630 was reflected in Dr Antonio Pellicini's recommendations to the Health Board in his treatise describing the initial stages of the epidemic:

> and remove those people shut up in houses, and especially the narrow evil shacks where there are a number of people living, not so much because of the many disorders which can take place, but because the enclosed air cannot be cleansed and is insalubrious.[47]

In August 1630 the Health Board was especially sensitised to the relationship between disease and smelly environments, as can be seen from the report of a corporal employed by the magistracy of the Otto on the 8 August:

> we passed near the house of Signor Lucha Salviati and smelling a great stink in Piazza de' Donati, which is near-by . . . we found nineteen barrels of excrement.[48]

They had begun to empty a cesspit and evidently, they had left it uncovered. This vigilance was taken one step further later in the month when it was decided by the Sanità to make a systematic investigation through instituting a sanitary survey. This built on a practice established by the Sanità from the late sixteenth century when medical men were sent to places infected by an epidemic to gather information about the sanitary conditions of the area, to describe the diseases of the sick and dead, and to determine the cause of the outbreak.[49] Even more urgent was when there were epidemics in the city, as during the outbreak of typhus in Florence in 1620–1621, when members of the charitable confraternity, the Buonomini di S. Martino, with doctors elected by the Sanità, instituted an inspection of the houses of the sick poor and found there 'a smell and fetor so great and insupportable'. So struck were they, that they commissioned a government official Filippo Lasagnini, responsible for the condition of Florence's streets, to undertake a thorough visit of the city and especially of the poorer areas. His description of the appalling insanitary conditions left the Sanità to conclude that 'proceeding in this way it is a miracle that it does not lead to a plague'.[50]

These were to prove portentous words when plague broke out in summer 1630 and the link between poverty and disease was acknowledged immediately, as recorded by Mario Guiducci in his *Panegyric* to the Grand Duke, written during the plague:

> they addressed the extreme misery of the poor, who languish in their houses, wasted away and in a sorry plight, not so much for their lack of food, as they have to sleep in beds which are so wretched, that it would be less troublesome to sleep in the places where unclean animals live like beasts.[51]

Following the practice of 1620–1621, a survey was implemented of the whole city, concentrating on the poorest streets: 'These [miserable beds] were to be carried away, the houses of the poor were to be cleansed from this dirt, and proper mattresses should be substituted in place of the vile piles of straw and the wretched rags'.[52] As in 1620–1621, the survey was delegated by the Sanità to the members of a religious confraternity, in this case, the Company of S. Michele Arcangelo, which had fulfilled this task on behalf of the city from the early sixteenth century.[53] The brief of the Company was to concentrate on identifying any problems associated with the systems for dealing with cesspits and the distribution of drinking water as well as with inadequate or defective bedding.[54]

The surviving copy of the survey, initiated on 10 August, records the genuine concern of the *confratelli* over the living conditions of the poor, hardly surprising since many members were nobles from the Grand-Ducal court. This was a very detailed investigation with the brothers going from house to house and indeed from apartment to apartment, mounting stairs, going through smelly courtyards and into equally smelly basements, to investigate the cause of odours emanating from leaking or over-full cesspits and drains. As Nicholas Eckstein has shown recently, the survey can be thought of as a type of 'walking map', in which the *Gentilomini* (Gentlemen or *Visitatori*) walked the streets of the city and identified individuals and places 'not by a specific address, but by spatial relationships that weave physical movement into the fabric of the Florentine urban environment'.[55]

Some idea of the number and distribution of these problems can be appreciated from an analysis of all cases of leaking cesspits and rotten mattresses listed in two major surveys in August in the largest parish in the city, S. Lorenzo.[56] The parish contained about 15 per cent of the city's population. It stretched from the centre, just north of the Baptistery, to the northern city walls at Porta San Gallo, and to the Fortezza da Basso in the north-west, and was characterised by a wide social and professional mix (see Figure 3.2). It also included a range of building types, from the patrician palaces in the centre to the complex of conventual and hospital buildings on Via S. Gallo, all linked together by the numerous streets of terraced houses inhabited by artisans and poorer folk. Just as morbidity and mortality rates were highest in the narrow streets with a high-density population, so were these sanitary problems. It was in these poorer streets that most of the 770 instances of problems associated with cesspits, water supply, and rotten mattresses were discovered during the surveys begun on 10 and 16 August. It is interesting that far more mattresses needed to be replaced (656) than cesspits requiring repair (114).

This is not unexpected given that every person living in these crowded houses would have needed a mattress or *paliasse* on which they slept, while there was usually no more than one cesspit per house, and in theory, it should have been repaired at the expense of the landlord.

Another important task assigned to the Gentlemen was not just to: 'remake straw mattresses and to remove filth', but also 'to take note of the sick that are found in the houses'.[57] There were variations in how much information was recorded for each section of the city, depending on how rigorously the Gentlemen fulfilled their task. Thus the Sesto of S. Croce provided much more detail about the health of the inhabitants than did those surveying the Sesto of S. Giovanni, noting, for example, cases of 'fever, catarrh, malattie di spine'.[58] This was reinforced by the Sanità, who passed a decree on 27 August giving instructions to the brothers that when they visited the parishes of the city, they should make a note of the 'symptoms [*accidenti*] of the sick', and send this information to the chancellor of the Sanità; at the same time it was emphasised to all heads of household that it was their duty, under threat of punishment, to report any sick person in their houses.[59] The close association between poverty and disease in the minds of the *Gentilomini* is clearly reflected in the entry about Agnolo di Francesco, who lived between Canto alle Macine and S. Lorenzo; he is described as 'sick from suffering and fever'.[60]

The houses of the poor were not confined to the backstreets, as can be seen from the following account of the inhabitants of the medieval tower at the Canto alla Paglia (see Figure 3.3), which was opposite the Baptistery of S. Giovanni, on the corner of Borgo S. Lorenzo and Via dei Carnesechi (now Via Cerretani). Particular attention would have been paid to this building because the apartments were above a shop belonging to a butcher, an occupation which in itself would have been seen as creating pollution through the release of the corrupt vapours contained in bodies of animals when they were slaughtered and cut up.[61] The tower was divided into four separate apartments, each with problems of its own:

> on the first floor of the said tower: to the widow Monna Lisa a new straw mattress; climbing another staircase: to Monna Lisabetta, wife of Bartolommeo Porta, another mattress; to Francesca on the said floor: mend a cesspit.
>
> On the top floor: a straw mattress to Andrea the tailor; and instruct the landlord of the said [apartment], who is the above-mentioned Moscellaro, to have carried away all the rubbish in the said house because it causes a great stink.
>
> The house which is built next door: to the son of the widow, the stretcher-bearer: a new straw mattress and empty the well; the landlord of it is called il Grazzini.[62]

This description, then, follows the journey of the inspector from the ground to the top floor in what were probably quite cramped apartments, or even individual rooms in a medieval tower. Like others built from the thirteenth

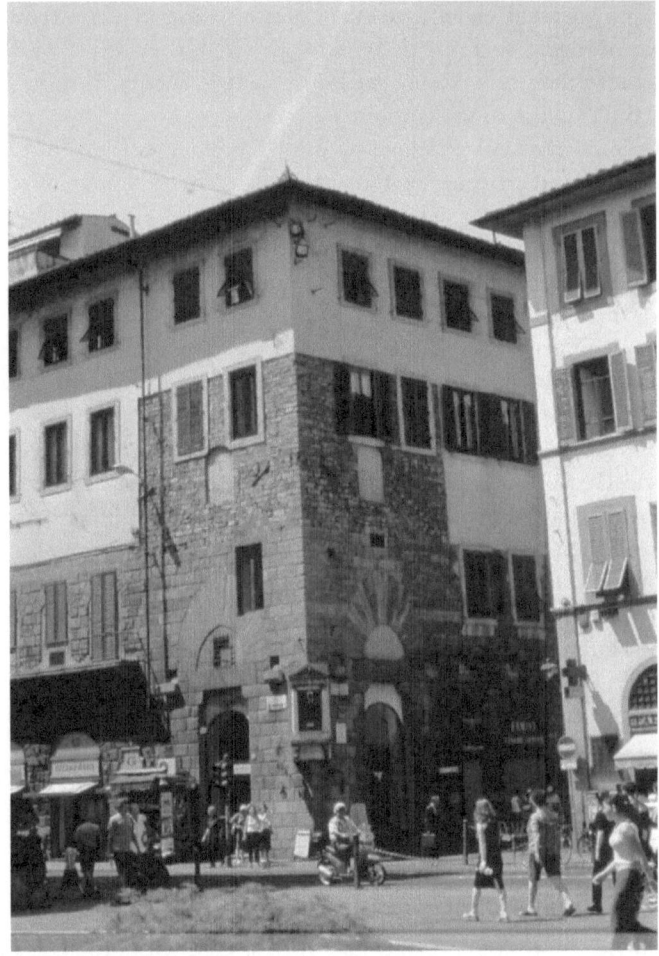

**FIGURE 3.3**  Canto alla Paglia, Florence. Author photo

century onwards, they were tall narrow buildings with sometimes no more than one or two rooms per floor, as is suggested by the official having had to climb the staircase from Monna Lisa's room to those of Monna Lisabetta and Monna Francesca. Even though this extract from the Company's visit is brief, it has enabled us to determine some of the characteristics which contemporaries saw as constituting 'the poor', and in turn how their living conditions were seen as reflecting that poverty. First, this group of half a dozen people were all living in rented accommodation in squalid conditions, with a landlord who was normally too mean to have the rubbish cleared away. In this, and the house next door, there were also problems with either the supply of clean water or the system to deal with human waste. We know that two of these women were widows, presumably living in straightened circumstances. They are represented as being too poor to buy decent mattresses; their own were seen as harbouring the poison of disease. Finally, two of the men would have been regarded as potentially suspect within the context of plague, Andrea the tailor and the stretcher-bearer, the first because he dealt with cloth and the second because he came into contact with the sick.

The emphasis in this passage, as in the rest of the survey, was on poverty and insanitary conditions, which often met in the same house. Over and again during this survey, the Gentlemen encountered widows or women living by themselves in abject poverty. In this case, the level of indigence was measured by the lack of bedding. Some such as Monna Fiore, the widow of Camillo the cobbler of Via S. Gallo, was found sleeping on the floor, as did the five women tenants further down the street and the weaver Lisabetta di Tommaso with her five children in Via Campaccio.[63]

In other cases, the precarious economic climate had led to the splitting up of families, as with Maddalena di Giovanni, who was described as a twenty-four-year-old 'girl', who lived in Via dell'Amore next to Piccini the baker. She also slept on the floor and was to be given a *paliasse*, although this was not enough to supply her needs, since she is described as having been abandoned by her father and was subsequently sent to the beggars' hostel of the Mendicanti.[64] In Borgo S. Jacopo there lived a woman called Nannina with seven children; the family was in abject poverty, and they were described as 'dying of hunger'. The main bread-winner of the family, her husband Matteo Pallini, had been in Pisa for several months, possibly in search of work, and may very well have found it difficult to return with the restrictions placed on travellers during plague. Obviously, with such a large family, she would have found it difficult, if not impossible, to work and hence her parlous financial state.[65]

Evidently, whole houses were often divided up into letting rooms, which were desolate in their poverty, as:

> in the courtyard inside the Portaccia [in Via dell'Ariento] there are many wretched rooms with ten tenants, all unhappy: supply ten [new] paliasses and have everything burnt; they do not have any kind of sheet or cover; and [we] have carried away many mounds of rubbish that corrupt the air.[66]

When the Sanità received this report on the 'houses of the poor people of the city', they recorded their satisfaction with the 'diligence employed and the charity of those who had undertaken [the survey]'. They declared, moreover, that they would request the Grand Duke to provide subsidies to the poor and that those houses in greatest need were to be cleansed. However, charity was not provided for all; the Sanità requested a note of those poor people who were able to work in the woollen or silk trades and they were not given alms.[67]

Two of the main aims of the survey had thus been achieved, to establish the extent of the needs of the poor and the extent of those insanitary conditions which might generate disease and help to create an epidemic.

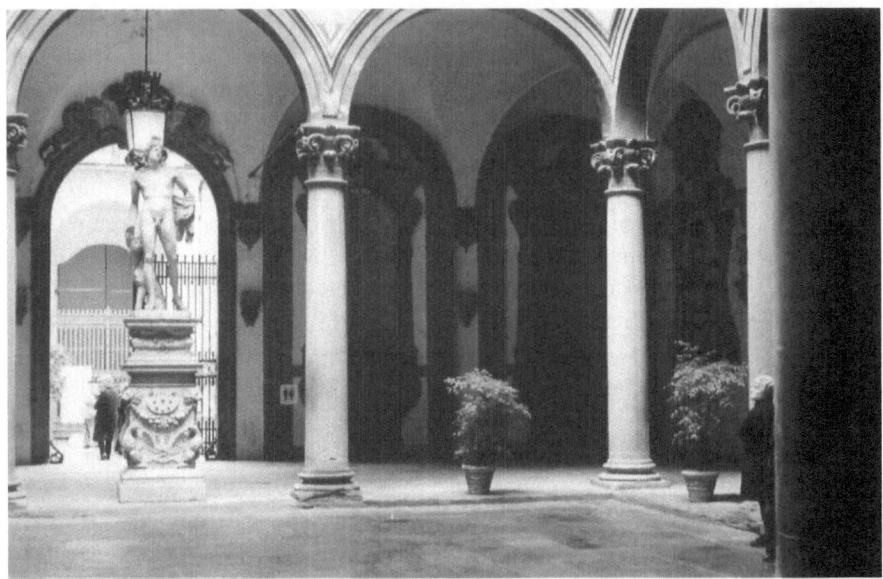

**FIGURE 3.4**  Courtyard of the Palazzo Medici-Riccardi, Florence. Author photo

This concern for filth, smells, and corrupt air can be seen even more graphically in a scene which was probably not uncommon in early modern cities, but in more normal times might not have been the cause of such alarm. The circumstances were ultimately the responsibility of the Grand Dukes because they were caused by workmen in Palazzo Medici, which remained their property, even though the family had taken up residence in Palazzo Pitti (see Figure 3.4):

> in the courtyard of the Palazzo de' Medici where the labourers are working on the chapel there are the common places which give off the most terrible stink in the whole street, and the same is true under the portico and where the labourers live, therefore they should be reconstructed in other places which are properly ventilated.[68]

Problems arose when provision had to be made for builders working on a property, either because they were lazy or because the proprietor did not allow access to their own toilets. The Medici Grand Dukes were also ultimately responsible for a similar problem for their employees:

> in the stables of the Grand Duke: mend the common place in Adam's room and also the sink because they create a great stink, and take away the rubbish and the filth from a hole where everybody throws things inside.[69]

The Medici were not the only landowners whose property created insanitary conditions, as can be seen in the case of the nuns of S. Orsola, for in the road behind their convent 'there is a drain leading from the water-troughs where the nuns work; twice a week all the stinking water runs out, which infects the street'.[70] The brothers ordered that the drain should be covered or a well should be dug, which would drain off the water from the trough. A major reason for these problems was the difficulty in establishing who was responsible for drains once wastewater had left the premises, the landlord or institution or the city, and then enforcing the regulations. In Via Panicale, for example, the *Gentilomini* ordered that a drain should be repaired because it 'receives the [water from] the washrooms of twelve houses at the back'.[71] In the case of a house near Canto alle Macine inhabited by the patrician Tommaso Pandolfini, 'there is a drain that discharges into the street and causes the greatest stink', so the landlord Piero, the olive oil dealer, is ordered to construct a well to collect the fetid water.[72] But tenants could also be the cause of the problem, as in another house near Canto alle Macine, where orders were issued to 'all the tenants who wash their clothes or other things, that they should not wash them in the house so that the stinking water does not find its way into the street'.[73]

The system to deal with the human waste of tenants could also be defective, as was reflected in the case of the medieval tower at the Canto alla Paglia and numerous other entries in these surveys, such as in the house in the Sestiere of S. Ambrogio between Via Nuova and Borgo Pinti, cited at the beginning of this chapter, where the tenants 'do everything in the same courtyard'.[74] While legislation and medical reports may have put the blame for filthy living conditions firmly on the shoulders of the poor, many entries in the sanitary survey underline that it was the responsibility of the landlord to provide the sanitary facilities involving not just latrines, but also the provision of fresh water and the disposal of all sorts of waste generated within the domestic context. Clearly one of the most problematic areas within houses were the cellars, partly because this is where the cesspits (*pozzi neri*) were often situated, as in the case of two houses in Via S. Zanobi, one rented by Francesco Perugino, where the contents of the cesspit was 'filling' the cellar, and the other rented by Francesco di Lorenzo which 'has a ruined cesspit'.[75]

The cellar was also the place where pipes entered the property, whether for clean water supply, where this existed, or for drainage pipes linking to the channels for wastewater in the street, as can be seen from the following entry relating to the S. Ambrogio area, where rubbish had been dumped: 'No 21: At the Canto ai Leoni there is a cellar where in addition to being full of filth, a female dog has died there . . . one can smell the stink all around and many people are complaining'.[76] Here again one can see the association between filth (*porcheria*) and the fear of plague, made worse by the fact that a dead dog had been dumped there, which was clearly regarded as a health problem by the *Gentilomini* who surveyed the area and more generally by locals.

One of the reasons for the numerous problems with the *pozzi neri* may have been the recent change in the system. Until the early sixteenth century it had been the job of the *votapozzieri* (literally sewer-emptiers), who were paid by the state to empty the *pozzi neri* on a regular basis. They emptied the liquid matter into the Arno and sold the solid matter to the *contadini* to fertilise their fields.[77] Then in the early seventeenth century the proprietors and the *contadini* decided to bypass the *votapozzieri*, with property-owners selling the matter directly to the *contadini*. De-regulation, of course, led to problems since there was now no proper control of waste disposal and resulted in complaints about the stench of the Arno and the surrounding areas. A new law was passed in 1621 during the typhus epidemic to remedy this abuse so that in future only the officially appointed *votapozzieri* could deal with waste. However, when it was decreed that landlords had to foot the bill, some decided to get the tenants to pay instead, but, because the poorest could not afford it, the *pozzi* were left to overflow.[78]

The brothers of the Company of S. Michele Arcangelo understood well the association between stink and plague and must have been keenly aware of their own exposure to disease while they conducted their survey. Risks to their own health and to that of the city are clearly evident from this note on 30 August by one of the *Gentilomini*, Lionardo Ginori, when he made his survey of Via Chiara:

> in distributing the straw mattresses today we discovered that the household goods were being removed belonging to someone whom they say had died while he was being taken to the hospital. Having heard that it was a suspicious disease, I ordered that the said goods that they wanted to carry into another house should not be touched. It seemed good to me to give an account of this to Your Most Illustrious Lords, how I found a sick woman in the Stufa Vecchia of Via dell'Ariento and that the above- mentioned person who died lived opposite the baker of S. Bernaba.[79]

This report reflects the care which was taken by these men appointed to survey the city to trace the physical proximity of cases of sickness and to report any incidence of suspicious death. The report shows clearly how information was gathered as they made their way along the streets inspecting houses. Evidently, on discovering somebody taking goods out of a house, Ginori had interviewed neighbours, who had told him that the man had died on the way to hospital and that it was evidently a suspicious death. All these streets were in close proximity and it is possible that the dead woman had visited the baker opposite S. Bernaba where the man had died. Ginori would have known this area intimately since Palazzo Ginori, where his family lived, was around the corner; indeed one can almost hear his patrician voice asking the questions and eliciting answers – 'they say', 'having heard' – from the more humble people of his neighbourhood.

The brothers of the Company of San Michele who had been designated to carry out the survey were genuinely shocked by the poverty, filth, and stinking air caused by the living conditions of the poor; as they noted in their report on the Sesto di S. Maria Novella on 22 August:

and one sees in the poverty from one day to the next an increase in the miseries and infinite needs, and if you had wanted us to note every case we would have had to create a large volume indeed.[80]

By early September the Sanità records that a total of 2,347 straw mattresses had been handed out to the poor by the confraternity, equivalent to giving a mattress to 3 per cent of the resident population.[81]

Concern was expressed above all that these insanitary conditions would create and increase the corrupt vapours, which were seen as creating plague, for, as Rondinelli had put it, 'filth is the mother of corruption'.[82] However, even if the results of the sanitary surveys of late summer 1630 appear to have shocked the brothers who conducted them, they cannot have been that surprised, given their normal daily experience must have included encounters with areas of the city which gave off smells generated by both domestic and industrial waste. What impact the survey had on the longer-term sanitary conditions in the city is difficult to judge, given the similarity between these findings and the anonymous description in February 1631 during the quarantine of the city. Indeed this survey was followed by another in the following spring.[83] Although its aim was not to describe the sanitary conditions, it instead outlined the number of people living in poverty, who were in need of state subsidies to survive and, like the earlier survey, in the process, they identified those who were sick from plague and 'ordinary sicknesses'. Taken together these two surveys emphasise how far governments had come to identify poverty, disease, and the urban environment, and, while outbreaks of epidemic disease may have concentrated their minds, it should not be forgotten that these measures were also part of a long tradition of sanitary legislation.

## Conclusion

One of the themes of this chapter has been the relationship between the better-off and the poor. However, for the most part, the records discussed, including laws, medical treatises, and sanitary surveys, reflect a top-down perspective, rather than that of the poorer sections of society, who were often the objects of government policy. These sources frequently reflected prejudices regarding the behaviour and living conditions of the poor, used to justify what appear to have been quite draconian measures to keep the poor in their places through systems of quarantine and punishment. However, this was not simply a question of social opposition; reality was much more complex. Thus the reactions of the brothers of the Company of S. Michele reveal genuine compassion in their visits to the poorer streets. It is also too easy from our perspective to condemn the insanitary conditions revealed by the survey, for even to have instituted it reflects a considerable awareness of these problems in their city and the necessity to remedy the situation. This speaks to a desire to improve the living conditions of the poor, a movement which was emphasised by the neo-Hippocratic revival, which placed emphasis on the close association between the urban environment, health and disease.

## Notes

1 Rondinelli, *Relazione*, 24. I am grateful to Yale University Press for permission to publish the material in this chapter, which forms part of my forthcoming monograph, provisionally entitled *Florence under Siege*.
2 Archivio di Stato di Firenze (cited as ASF), Compagnie religiose soppresse da Pietro Leopoldo (CRS), 1418.6.A, no.3, f. 2v. This chapter emerges out of the ESRC-funded project, 'Epidemics and Mortality in the Pre-Industrial City: Florence and London Compared', from 1989 to 1992. Discussed in Henderson, 'Public Health, Pollution and the Problem of Waste Disposal, 373–382; in more detail in Henderson, *Florence under Siege*, Chapter 8. See also Eckstein, 'Florence on Foot', 1–25, whose 'specific concern is with the *Visita* as a city survey', complementary to my own work on the history of public health.
3 See Pellicini, *Discorso*.
4 De Castro, *Il curioso*, 15.
5 *Ibid.*, 19.
6 Henderson, 'The Black Death in Florence', 142.
7 Geltner, 'Healthscaping', 395–415.
8 Cipolla, *Miasmas and Disease*, on late sixteenth-century surveys of Tuscany; Cohn, *Cultures of Plague*, Chapter 7; Wear, 'Making Sense of Health'.
9 See, for example, Rawcliffe, *Urban Bodies*.
10 *Cf.* Riley, *The Eighteenth-Century Campaign to Avoid Disease*.
11 Cohn, *Cultures of Plague*, 202–207.
12 This built on an existing tradition; see for the preceding period: Carmichael, *Plague and the Poor*.
13 For a comparison between policies towards plague and the Great Pox see: Henderson, 'Coping with Plagues in Renaissance Italy', 175–194; Arrizabalaga, Henderson, and French, *The Great Pox*. See also Cohn, *Cultures of Plague*, 7; see also Stevens-Crawshaw, *Plague Hospitals*.
14 Terpstra, *Cultures of Charity*.
15 Cohn, *Cultures of Plague*, 227–229.
16 Pullan, 'Plague and Perceptions of the Poor', 101–123.
17 Henderson, '"La schifezza, madre di corruzione"', 23–56.
18 Del Panta, *Le epidemie*, 160, Table 24.
19 Studies of the 1630–1631 plague in Florence range from Lombardi's study '(1629–1631): crisi e peste a Firenze', 3–50 to Lichfield, *Florence Ducal Capital*, Chapter 7, though Calvi, *Histories*, remains the most detailed study, based on the court cases brought against those who broke the plague decrees of the Health Board during the epidemic.
20 For Italy see: Carmichael, 'Plague Legislation', 208–225; 'Contagion Theory and Contagion Practice, 213–256; Benvenuto, *La peste nell'Italia della prima età moderna*, and most recently 'Le retour de la peste'.
21 Outlined most recently in Henderson, '"La schifezza, madre di corruzione"'.
22 On the role of the Misericordia see: Henderson, 'Plague in Renaissance Florence', 165–186.
23 *Cf.* Fosi (ed.), *La Peste a Roma (1656–1657)*.
24 For the earlier period see: Carmichael, *Plague and the Poor*.
25 Cohn, *Cultures of Plague*, Chapter 7.
26 *Cf.* Cavallo and Storey, *Healthy Living*.
27 On early modern England see: Wear, *Knowledge and Practice*, 184–209.
28 Rondinelli, *Relazione*, 26–27.
29 See Cipolla, *I pidocchi e il Granduca*.

30 Rondinelli *Relazione*, 30, 40; *Cf.* Righi, *Historia*, 23–26, on diet; *Cf.* Pullan, 'Plague and Perceptions of the Poor', 108–110. For similar sentiments expressed by medical writers in early modern England see: Wear, *Knowledge and Practice*, 281–286.

31 Righi, *Historia*; De Castro, *Il curioso*.

32 Righi, *Historia*, 17; De Castro, *Il curioso*, 9.

33 De Castro, *Il curioso*, 9.

34 *Ibid.*; *Cf.* discussion by Calvi, *Histories of a Plague Year*, 64–65.

35 Righi, *Historia*, 11–12.

36 Pastore, *Crimine e giustizia in tempo di peste*, 188.

37 Lombardi, *Povertà maschile, Povertà femminile*.

38 Rondinelli, *Relazione*, 25.

39 *Ibid.*, 34, 44–46. See also discussion in Lombardi, '(1629–1631): crisi e peste a Firenze'; Lichfield, *Florence Ducal Capital*, Chapter 7; and see Henderson and Rose, 'Plague and the City', Chapter 7.

40 Rondinelli, *Relazione*, 34, 44–46.

41 See Henderson, *Florence under Siege*, Chapter 8 (forthcoming), for a detailed discussion of actual punishments given to those breaking the Health Board's decrees.

42 The subject of: Calvi, *Histories of a Plague Year*, and also Henderson, *Florence under Siege*, Chapter 8; See Lichfield, *Florence Ducal Capital*, on the economic background.

43 ASF, Sanità, Negozi 155, ff. 259r–v: undated, *c.* 8 February 1631.

44 *Ibid.*

45 Cipolla, *Miasmas and Disease*; Cipolla, *I pidocchi*; Eckstein, 'Florence on Foot', 19–20

46 Brighetti, *Bologna e la peste del 1630*, 38–39; Sansa, 'Strategie di prevenzione a confronto', 93–109; Gentilcore, 'Purging Filth', 153–168.

47 Pellicini, *Discorso*, 14.

48 ASF, Sanità, Negozi 150, f 405r: 8.viii.30.

49 See Cipolla, *Miasmas and Disease*.

50 Cipolla, *Miasmas and Disease*, 13–14; ASF, Sanità 138, f. 1058r: 3.i.1621.

51 Guiducci, 'Panegirico', in: Rondinelli, *Relazione*, 124.

52 *Ibid.* The survey is in: ASF, Compagnie Religiose Soppresse da Pietro Leopoldo (CRS), 1418.

53 *Cf.* Eckstein, 'Florence on Foot', on the history and membership of this confraternity.

54 ASF, Sanità, Copialettere 55, f. 102r.

55 Eckstein, 'Florence on Foot', 18.

56 See Henderson and Rose, 'Plague and the City', to be further developed in Henderson, *Florence under Siege*.

57 ASF, CRS, 1418.6 A.II, no.12.

58 *Ibid.*, no.7.

59 ASF, Sanità, Decreti e Partiti 6, f. 80r: 28.viii.1630.

60 ASF, CRS, 1418.6 A.II, no. 206: 16.viii.1631.

61 Cipolla, *Miasmas and Disease*, 23, 64. *Cf.* Zagli *et al.*, *Maladetti beccari*. Legislation against butchers was a recurrent theme of medieval sanitary legislation; *Cf.* Henderson, 'The Black Death in Florence', 143, and Rawcliffe, Chapter 1, this volume.

62 ASF, CRS, 1418.6A.II, nos. 210–212.

63 *Ibid.*, A.9: unpaginated, but identified by location: 'a Chiarito' and 'Nel Campaccio no. 8'.

64 ASF, CRS, 1418.6A.15: unpaginated, but identified by location and date: 13.viii.30.

65 *Ibid.*: unpaginated, but identified by location and date: 22.viii.30.

66 *Ibid.*, no. 64.

67 *Ibid.*, dated 19.viii.1630

68 *Ibid.*, no. 220.

69 *Ibid.*, f 6r: no. 20.

70 *Ibid.*, f 6r, no. 112: 16.viii.30.

71 ASF, CRS, 1418.11, no. 15: 16.viii.1630.

72 *Ibid.*, no. 207: 16.viii.1630.

73  *Ibid.*, no. 205.
74  *Ibid.*, 1418.6.A, no. 3, f. 2v.
75  *Ibid.*, CRS, 1418.6. no. 9, under Via S. Zanobi.
76  ASF, CRS, 1418.6A, ff. 6r–v: no. 21.
77  See: Cipolla, *I pidocchi e il Granduca*, 60–67; Henderson, 'Public Health, Pollution and the Problem of Waste Disposal'.
78  *Ibid.*
79  Sanità 150, f. 1572r: 30.viii.1630.
80  ASF, CRS, 1418.6A, Sestiere of Santa Maria Novella, no.15: 22.viii.1630.
81  Sanità 151, f. 53r:2.ix.1630.
82  Rondinelli, *Relazione*, 24.
83  For example, Sanità 465: Sestiere di S. Spirito.

# References

## Archival sources

All archival records cited are in the Archivio di Stato di Firenze (ASF).

Compagnie Religiose Soppresse da Pietro Leopoldo, 1418.6: Aug.–Sept. 1630.

Ufficiali di Sanità, Copialettere 55 (June–Oct. 1630).

Ufficiali di Sanità, Decreti e Partiti 6 (June–Oct. 1630).

Ufficiali di Sanità, Negozi, 138 (1618–1620), 150 (Aug. 1630), 151 (Sept. 1630), 155 (Feb.– March 1631).

Ufficiali di Sanità, 465: 'Descrizione delle case e delle persone', Sesto di Santo Spirito, census during the quarantine of the city, Jan. 1631.

## Printed primary sources

De Castro, Stefano Roderico, *Il curioso nel quale dialogo si discorre del male di peste* (Pisa: Francesco Tanagli, 1631).

Guiducci, Mario, 'Panegirico al serenissimo Ferdinando II Duca di Toscana per la liberazione di Firenze della peste', in: Francesco Rondinelli, *Relazione del contagio stato in Firenze l'anno 1630 e 1633* (Florence: Landini, 1634).

Pellicini, Antonio, *Discorso sopra di mali contagiosi pestilenziali* (Florence: Zanobi Pignoni, 1630).

Righi, Alexandro, *Historia contagiosi morbi qui Florentiniam popolatus fuit anno 1630* (Florence, Francesco Onofrio, 1633).

Rondinelli, Francesco, *Relazione del contagio stato in Firenze l'anno 1630 e 1633* (Florence: Landini, 1634).

## Printed secondary sources

Arrizabalaga, Jon, John Henderson, and Roger French, *The Great Pox: The French Disease in Renaissance Europe* (New Haven, CT and London: Yale University Press, 1997).

Benvenuto, Graziella, *La peste nell'Italia della prima età moderna. Contagio, rimedi, profilassi* (Bologna: CLUEB, 1995).

Brighetti, Antonio, *Bologna e la peste del 1630* (Bologna: Aulo Gaggi, 1968).

Calvi, Giulia, *Histories of a Plague Year: The Social and Imaginary in Baroque Florence* (Berkeley and Los Angeles: California University Press, 1989).

Carmichael, Ann G., 'Contagion Theory and Contagion Practice in Fifteenth-Century Milan', *Renaissance Quarterly*, 42 (1991), 213–256.

Carmichael, Anne G., *Plague and the Poor in Renaissance Florence* (Cambridge, UK: Cambridge University Press, 1986).

Carmichael, Anne G., 'Plague Legislation in the Italian Renaissance', *Bulletin of the History of Medicine*, 57, 4 (1983), 208–225.

Cavallo, Sandra, and Storey, Tessa, *Healthy Living in Late Renaissance Italy* (Oxford: Oxford University Press, 2013).

Cipolla, Carlo M., *I pidocchi e il Granduca. Crisi economica e problemi sanitari nella Firenze del '600* (Bologna: Il Mulino, 1979).

Cipolla, Carlo M., *Miasmas and Disease: Public Health and the Environment in the Pre-Industrial Age* (New Haven, CT and London: Yale University Press, 1992).

Cohn, Samuel K., *Cultures of Plague: Medical Thinking at the End of the Renaissance* (Oxford: Oxford University Press, 2010).

Del Panta, Lorenzo, *Le epidemie nella storia demografica italiana (secoli XIX–XIX)* (Turin: Loescher, 1980).

Eckstein, Nicholas A., 'Florence on Foot: An Eye-level Mapping of the Early Modern City in Time of Plague', *Renaissance Studies*, 30, 2 (2016), 1–25.

Fosi, Irene (ed.), *La Peste a Roma (1656–1657)* (Rome: Università Roma Tre-CROMA, 2006).

Geltner, Guy, 'Healthscaping a Medieval City: Lucca's *Curia viarum* and the Future of Public Health History', *Urban History*, 40, 3 (2015), 395–415.

Gentilcore, David, 'Purging Filth: Plague and Responses to it in Rome, 1656–1657', in: Mark Bradley and Kenneth Stow (eds.), *Rome, Pollution and Propriety: Dirt, Disease and Hygiene in the Eternal City from Antiquity to Modernity* (Cambridge, UK, Cambridge University Press, 2012), 153–168.

Henderson, John, 'Plague in Renaissance Florence: Medical Theory and Government Response', in: Neithard Bulst and Robert Delort (eds.), *Maladies et société (xii–xviii siècles)* (Paris: Editions du CNRS, 1989), 165–186.

Henderson, John, '"La schifezza, madre di corruzione": Peste e società a Firenze nella prima epoca moderna', *Medicina e Storia*, 2 (2001), 23–56.

Henderson, John, *Florence under Siege. Surviving the Plague in a Seventeenth-Century City.* (New Haven, CT and London: Yale University Press), forthcoming.

Henderson, John, 'Public Health, Pollution and the Problem of Waste Disposal in Early Modern Tuscany', in: Simonetta Cavaciocchi (ed.), *Le interazioni fra economia e ambiente biologico nell'Europa preindustriale, secc. XIII–XVIII* (Florence: Firenze University Press, 2010), 373–382.

Henderson, John, 'The Black Death in Florence: Medical and Communal Responses', in: Steven Bassett (ed.), *Death in Towns: Urban Responses to the Dying and the Dead, 100–1600* (Leicester: Leicester University Press, 1992), 136–150.

Henderson, John and Colin Rose, 'Plague and the City: Methodological Considerations in Mapping Disease in Early Modern Florence', in: Nicholas Terpstra and Colin Rose (eds.), *Mapping Space, Sense, and Movement in Florence* (London: Routledge, 2016), 125–146.

Henderson, John, 'Coping with Plagues in Renaissance Italy', in: Linda Clark, and Carole Rawcliffe (eds.), *The Fifteenth Century XII, Society in an Age of Plague* (Woodbridge: Boydell and Brewer, 2013), 175–194.

Lichfield, Burr, *Florence Ducal Capital, 1530–1630* (New York: ACLS Humanities E-Book, c. 2008).

Lombardi, Daniela, '(1629–1631): crisi e peste a Firenze', *Archivio storico italiano*, cxxxvii, 1979, 3–50.

Lombardi, Daniela, *Povertà maschile, Povertà femminile. L'Ospedale dei Mendicanti nella Firenze dei Medici* (Bologna: Il Mulino, 1988).

Pastore, Alessandro, *Crimine e giustizia in tempo di peste nell'Europa moderna* (Roma-Bari: La Terza, 1991).

Pullan, Brian, 'Plague and Perceptions of the Poor in Early Modern Italy', in: T. Ranger and P. Slack (eds.), *Epidemics and Idea:. Essays on the Historical Perception of Pestilence* (Cambridge, UK: Cambridge University Press, 1992), 101–123.

Rawcliffe, Carole, *Urban Bodies. Communal Health in Late Medieval English Towns and Cities* (Woodbridge: Boydell Press, 2013).

'Le retour de la peste. Nouvelles recherches sur les épidémies en Europe et en Méditerranée xive-xixe siècles', in: *Annales de Demographie Historique*, 2 (2017).

Riley, James C., *The Eighteenth-Century Campaign to Avoid Disease* (Basingstoke: Macmillan, 1987).

Sansa, Renato, 'Strategie di prevenzione a confronto l'igiene urbana durante la peste romana del 1656–1657' in: Irene Fosi (ed), *La Peste a Roma (1656–1657),* (Rome: Università Roma Tre-CROMA, 2006), 93–109.

Stevens-Crawshaw, Jane, *Plague Hospitals: Public Health for the City in Early Modern Venice* (Ashgate: Farnham, 2012).

Terpstra, Nicholas, *Cultures of Charity: Women, Politics, and the Reform of Poor Relief in Renaissance Italy* (Cambridge, MA: Harvard University Press, 2013).

Wear, Andrew, *Knowledge and Practice in English Medicine, 1550–1680* (Cambridge, UK: Cambridge University Press, 2000).

Wear, Andrew, 'Making Sense of Health and the Environment in Early Modern England', in: Andrew Wear (ed.), *Health and Healing in Early Modern England* (Aldershot: Ashgate, 1998), 119–147

Zagli, Andrea, Francesco Mineccia, Andrea Giuntini, *Maladetti beccari: storia dei macellari fiorentini dal Cinquecento al Duemila* (Florence: Polistampa, 2000).

# 4

# PLAGUE VIEWS

## Epidemics, photography, and the ruined city

*Robert Peckham*

### Introduction: the imperial album

The megacities that have mushroomed in the People's Republic of China with market liberalisation from the 1980s are often depicted in the global media as polluted, singularly unhealthy places. Urban expansion as a result of rural-to-city migration, dense living conditions, lax regulation, and the environmental fallout of fast-paced industrialisation are understood to be drivers of infectious disease. The emergence in Guangdong Province of avian influenza (H5N1) in 1996–1997 and severe acute respiratory syndrome (SARS) in 2002–2003 – the first 'plague' of the twenty-first century – are taken to exemplify the pandemic threat posed by China's urban conurbations and their ecological effects.[1] Today, booming cities, such as Shenzhen and Guangzhou, are represented as places of teeming crowds, wet markets and clean-up operations, anonymous tower blocks and quarantines, masked citizens and police checkpoints.[2] They are also evoked as agglomerations of disconcertedly deserted transit zones or 'non-places': 'haunting, empty commercial spaces such as airports, hotel lobbies, and convention centres'.[3] Relinquished of traffic, these ghost cities are conjured as hubs of disease manufacture and distribution, symptoms of a global system in reverse.[4] As Priscilla Wald has observed in relation to the news coverage of SARS: 'Guangdong exports disease as a commodity in the dangerously promiscuous spaces of a global economy conceived as an ecology'.[5]

This chapter traces the modern iconography of the plagued city back to late nineteenth-century Western depictions of Qing China, and in so doing investigates the co-evolution of urban, public health, and photographic technologies. As the sociologists Syed Harris Ali and Roger Keil remarked some time ago, 'not much specific work has been published on the urban aspects of emerging infectious diseases, particularly in the increasingly significant context of globalising cities and the global cities network'.[6] Taking up the challenge presented by this research lacuna, three interrelated questions are addressed that pivot on the connections between epidemics, the development of photography, and an expanding urban milieu. Under what conditions did the Chinese city figure in the global media as a locus of epidemic crisis? How has photography shaped the urban identity of disease? And in what ways have epidemics determined the development of urban photography? To answer these questions, the chapter brings together two major but often disconnected strands of research: a growing scholarship on photography and the city, and a burgeoning literature on the role of the visual and its apparatuses within medicine and public health.[7]

Notwithstanding this interest in biomedicine as a visual regime, surprisingly little has been written about photographic representations of infectious disease. As Christos Lynteris has recently observed: 'epidemic photography is a genre largely unexamined by visual studies, visual anthropology or indeed historians of medicine'.[8] Photographic visualisations of Chinese 'wet markets' during the SARS outbreak, however, have been central to the construction of a pandemic narrative that identifies live animals markets as sites of highly pathogenic animal-to-human 'spillovers'.[9] Building upon this work, the argument presented in this chapter is that key elements of contemporary epidemic photography can be found in the visual archive generated by the 'third plague pandemic'.[10] By examining a corpus of plague photographs from the 1890s – namely the plague views produced in Hong Kong by David Knox Griffith (1841–1897), '[the] last of the distinguished European commercial photographers active in 19th century China' – the chapter demonstrates how images of the plagued city drew on a rich visual storehouse, including two recognisable and interrelated photographic genres: ruin and disaster photography.[11]

Griffith was a commercial photographer who produced a diverse body of photographic work that ranged from portraits and panoramas to ethnographic and 'documentary' pictures. An advertisement for Griffith's studio, placed in a tourist guide in 1893, announced that buyers could procure views of Hong Kong, Canton, Macao, the coast of China, and Formosa (Taiwan). Among the photographs on sale were pictures of Chinese life, school scenes, domestic scenes, and scenes of execution.[12] In this respect, Griffith's plague views are unlike those taken by military officers or consultant engineers: for example, the pictures by Captain C. Moss and F. B. Stewart of the plague in Bombay between 1896 and 1897, or the photographs of the 1900 plague outbreak in Sydney produced by George McCredie for the Public Works Department.[13] Griffith's photographs were advertised and sold to tourists, reproduced in newspapers and travel books, and publicly exhibited; they also acquired quasi-official authority as evidence of the colonial state's public health drive.

In Hong Kong, commercial photographers not only catered to the demand of tourists for scenic postcards and curios, they also provided news coverage and undertook contracted work for government departments. From the 1870s, photography was being employed routinely in state operations. Photographs were used to record visits by dignitaries, to chart the progress of public works, such as afforestation efforts across the colony, to assess the damage inflicted by typhoons, and to map the colony – playing a key role, for example, in defining the boundary of the New Territories when these were acquired by the British in 1898 on a 99-year lease from the Qing. While photographs accompanied departmental reports to the governor, the Colonial Office in London could also request photographs from the colonial administration to clarify the scope of government projects. Photography assumed an importance in population control: in the registration of prostitutes and for the issuance of chair and rickshaw licences, as well as for the identification of prisoners in Victoria Goal. In 1888, several thousand Chinese cargo boatmen went on strike over a government plan to introduce a licence requirement at 25 cents per annum, which included the mandatory provision of a photograph 'for the purpose of iden-tification'.[14] In the event, the government backed down and the condition was applied only to head boatmen. Such policies reflected a gathering impetus through the 1880s to keep a check on the flow of migrant labour. As Governor Sir Richard MacDonnell had put it in 1866, Hong Kong was becoming the destination for 'the migratory refuse of many millions of Chinese'.[15] Photography could function in this context as a means of fixing identities and establishing order.

Photography was also a popular pastime taken up by scientists, government officials, and medical missionaries. The line between professional and amateur photography blurred. While Alexandre Yersin took photographs on his travels in Indochina, in Hong Kong he produced photomicrographs of the plague bacilli, as well as views of the plagued city.[16] Other participants involved in the outbreak were keen amateur photographers, a case in point being the German physician Hermann Wittenberg who worked for the Basel Mission in Kayintschu (Meizhou) and arrived in Hong Kong in June 1894 to help with the anti-plague efforts there.[17]

The aim of this chapter is thus to resituate photographs of the third plague pandemic within the heterogeneity of the imperial album, highlighting the interconnections between different photographic types and modalities – the pho-tograph as instrument of state, as news medium, as personal testimony, and as hobby – in order to show how referents were reconfigured as one photographic genre re-coded another.[18] Put somewhat differently, the chapter traces the redis-tribution of meanings across modalities. It argues that identifying the 'plague view' as a distinct category necessarily involves a distorting de-contextualisation since such plague representations cannot be disassociated from the broader visual culture within which they were produced. Epidemic photography was, in other words, a profoundly hybrid genre.[19]

The chapter is organised in four sections. The first section provides a brief over-view of Western photography in China, before introducing Griffith's life and work and setting this in the context of the 'photography complex'.[20] The second section considers the ruin as a sub-genre of urban and architectural photography in China and shows how an interest in the ruined city overlapped with other strands of late nineteenth-century metropolitan photography. The focus in this section is on the instrumental use of photography in debates about slum clearance and as a means of documenting the vanishing pre-modern city that this demolition entailed. The third section examines the work of Griffith in greater detail, placing his plague views of Hong Kong within the context of his career as a commercial photographer in China. Connections are drawn between Griffith's representations of the 1894 outbreak and the various strands of urban and architectural photography outlined in section one, including 'the visual archive of ruination'.[21] In the conclusion, the implications of the chapter's central argument are further elaborated.

Epidemic photography was part of the nineteenth-century 'evidentiary crescendo' that brought together and recombined different species of urban photography.[22] Examining this process of visual recombination is crucial to understanding the operations of an incipient global media. It also suggests how colonial 'media templates' continue to define depictions of epidemics in urban hotspots of the non-Western world.[23] Although there is now a significant literature examining the rhetorical manoeuvres of the 'outbreak narrative' and the 'dramaturgical' shape of epidemic crises, there has been little emphasis on how representations of urban space act as visual cues in moments of disease crisis.[24] Reflecting on the role of photography in the construction of disease emergence – and specifically in the construction of an urban topography of infection – may shed light on how epidemics are understood in relation to a prehistory of traumatic events that carry potent visual associations.

## China and the 'photography complex'

Hong Kong was established as a British colony by the terms of the Treaty of Nanking (Nanjing), which followed the defeat of the Qing in the First Opium War (1839–1842).[25] Although administratively British, the port city was overwhelmingly Chinese. According to the 1901 census, out of a total population of 283,905, only 6,431 were European or American civilians.[26] Hong Kong was also closely connected to the cities of south-west China. It was a 'space of flow', serving as a Western gateway into China, while thousands of sojourning labourers routinely crossed the border into Hong Kong.[27] Meanwhile, the Great Power scramble for influence in the Qing Empire was accompanied by the introduction of photography, particularly from the 1850s.[28] A cartoon by 'Cham' (Amédée de Noé), which appeared in the French weekly magazine Le charivari in 1858, caricatured the increasingly important role played by photography in the 'opening up' of China. Foreign photographers are depicted in the sketch besieging the horrified Xianfeng Emperor with their cameras.[29]

Western conflict with China in the mid-century spurred an ambivalent interest in China and Chinese artefacts.[30] Images of Chinese monuments, landscapes, and people were widely reproduced and circulated in metropolitan newspapers and magazines. The Italian-born, naturalised British photographer Felice Beato (1832–1909) documented the final stages of the campaign by the Anglo-French expeditionary forces in the Second Opium War (1856–1860), taking pictures of the Yuanming Yuan (Summer Palace) before its demolition by Allied troops.[31] In the early twentieth century, photojournalism became crucial in disseminating information about China. The Boxer Uprising in 1900 intensified news coverage with images of ruined cityscapes – among them the striking stereographic panoramas by the American photographer James Ricalton (1844–1929).[32] The foreign occupation of the Forbidden City, built by the Ming dynasty in the fifteenth century, marked the culmination of this photographic penetration of imperial China.

Griffith's plague views are perhaps the most enduring images of the 1894 Hong Kong plague outbreak, which marked the onset of the plague's global diffusion from China. Indeed, they have become iconic, often standing in metonymically for the pandemic itself. Griffith died in Hong Kong in January 1897, after more than two decades in China.[33] Born in Dublin in around 1841, he had been employed at the fashionable Dickinson Brothers photographic studio on New Bond Street, London, in the 1860s. He subsequently worked as a portrait photographer in the provinces before emigrating to China. By 1872, he had joined the studio of the successful commercial photographer William Thomas Saunders in Shanghai (1832–1892).[34] And by 1878, he had moved to Hong Kong, where he assisted the well-known Chinese photographer Lai Afong (c. 1839–1890). Six years later, he was advertising his own studio in the colony. A notice in the *China Mail* in 1885 commended Griffith's 'tasteful photographic New Year's cards' and the 'choice collection of Hongkong views and characteristic scenes for display in the India and Colonial Exhibition'.[35]

An article on the plague in the *Illustrated London News* in July 1894 was accompanied by a Griffith photograph showing troops from the Shropshire Light Infantry burning rubbish hauled from Chinese houses in a street of Taipingshan, an area in the Western District of Hong Kong Island that was at the epicentre of the outbreak (Figure 4.1). An engraving based on a similar Griffith photograph appeared on the cover of the *Graphic* in August 1894, with a picture of the men's ward of the 'Glassworks' hospital illustrating an editorial on the plague inside.[36] A photographic series, *Views of the Plague* that included the 'Glassworks' image and twelve other plague scenes was advertised by Griffith at the beginning of July 1894.

Although widely circulated, Griffith's authorship of the plague photographs is often unacknowledged. When he is credited, the pictures are invariably lifted from the rest of his oeuvre and presented as 'incontestable pictorial evidence' of the colonial state's draconian response.[37] Myron Echenberg's history of the third plague pandemic, for example, contains two of Griffith's images with no reference to the photographer. The engraving of a photograph by Griffith from the *Graphic*, which depicts soldiers disinfecting houses and burning refuse, serves an illustrative function in the book; its meaning is determined by the plague narrative that frames it.[38] The photograph is construed as a documentary testimony of an historic event and read, in effect, 'as a message without a code'.[39]

This taken-for-granted documentary status of plague photography invites critical questions about the function of photography and its uses as a tool for historians. Rather than viewing photographs as illustrative of an historical event, we might consider the photograph itself as an object with a history. The focus, in other words, might shift onto the 'social biography of the image'.[40] For what purpose were plague

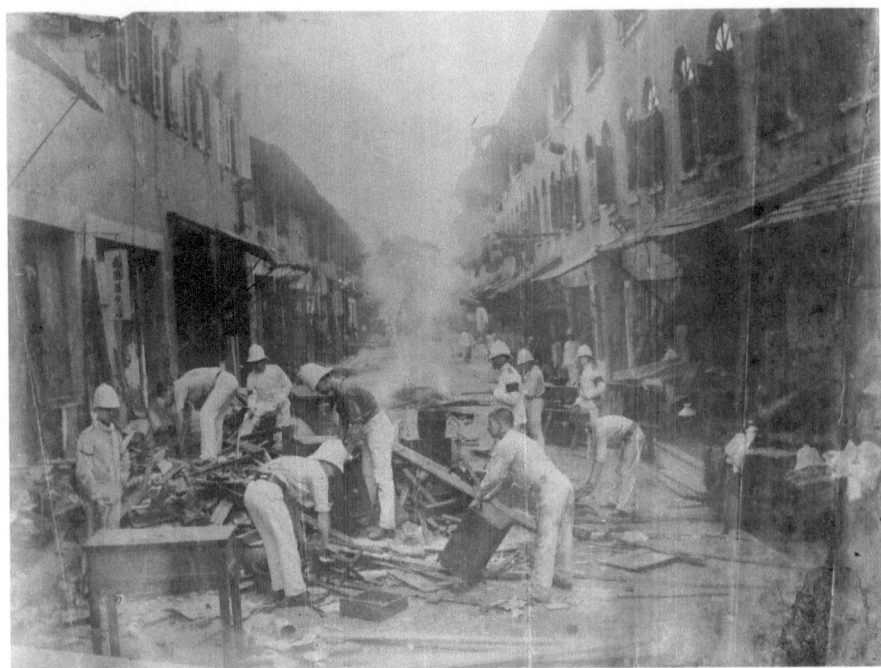

FIGURE 4.1   D. K. Griffith, 'Staffordshire regiment cleaning plague houses, Hong
Kong', 1894. A photograph from the plague series was reproduced in the
*Illustrated London News* (28 July 1894), 100. Source: Wellcome Library,
London

photographs produced? By whom and how were they used? What do they show?
As John Tagg has suggested 'every photograph is the result of specific and, in every
sense, significant distortions which render its relation to any prior reality deeply
problematic'.[41] To better understand these 'significant distortions', there is a need to
reconsider the multiple contexts that shaped photographic representations; in other
words, to view the plague images within a network of actants – 'the photography
complex' – that made their production and circulation possible.[42]

## 'A wilderness of ruin': catastrophic empire

From the 1860s, the Chinese 'ruin' as a sub-category of urban and architectural
photography was popularised in the work of Beato, Thomas Child (1841–1898),
John Thomson (1837–1921), Ernst Ohlmer (1847–1927), and others. As the art
historian, Wu Hung has suggested, nineteenth-century photographic images of
decaying Chinese buildings were part of 'the emergence of a transnational visual
culture of ruins in China'.[43] To be sure, the ruin-scape as a photographic subject was not confined to China. Beato had taken a 'portfolio of after-the-battle
images of death and ruin' in India during the Indian Rebellion (or 'Mutiny') of

1857 – one example being his picture of the gutted, body-strewn Sikandar Bagh Palace in Lucknow.[44] Similarly, Thomson's pictures of ruins in Cyprus taken in 1878, the year that the island became a British Protectorate under nominal Ottoman suzerainty, are reminiscent of his China oeuvre. The former were explicitly taken to 'afford a source of comparison in after years, when, under the influence of British rule, the place has risen from its ruins'.[45] Nonetheless, in a China context, the ruin was associated with the Qing Empire's 'opening up', with war reportage during a period of large-scale conflict that saw the Taiping Rebellion (1850–1864) – in which an estimated 20 million people perished – and the Second Opium War. At the same time, China ruin photography 'mixed western sentiment for decayed buildings, orientalistic fascination with "old China," and archaeological or ethnographic interests'.[46]

Beato's images of the 1860 Anglo-French campaign, for example, depict China as an empire in ruins. In his pictures of the Dagu Forts on the Hai River – strategic Chinese defences protecting Tianjin and the imperial capital, Peking (Beijing) – conflict has created an ambiguous space where inside and outside become indistinguishable. This is a shattered landscape of churned earth and half-demolished fortifications, where the strewn corpses of Chinese combatants merge disturbingly with the scattered debris (Figure 4.2).

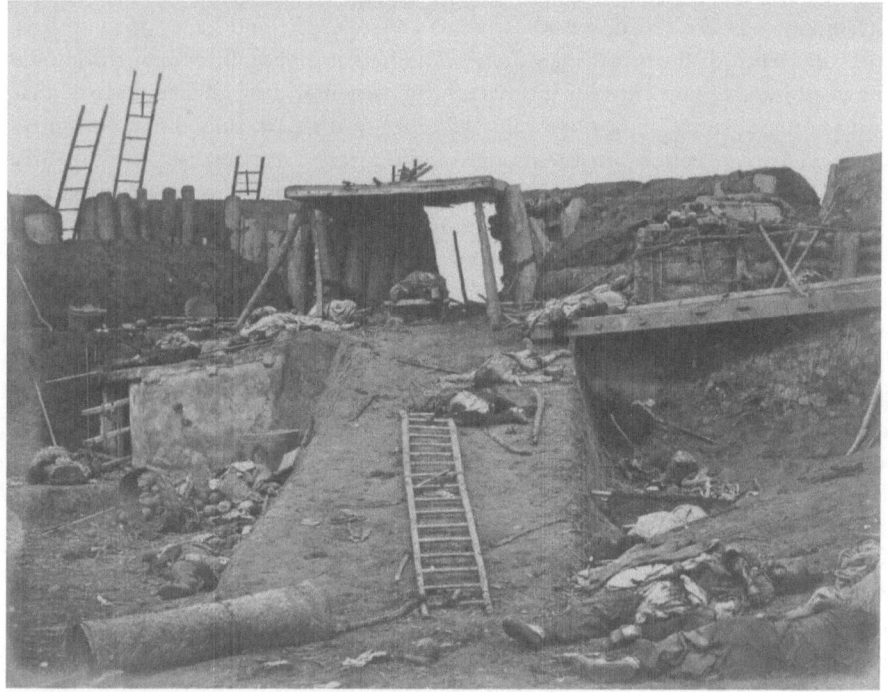

**FIGURE 4.2**  Felice Beato, 'Interior of the angle of North Fort', 21–22 August 1860.
Source: J. Paul Getty Museum, Los Angeles

There is a strikingly performative quality to this work, which envisions the battlefield as a stage set.[47] Like a natural disaster, war is dramatised obliquely. Beato's pictures capture the aftermath of a catastrophic impact that has evidently swept, typhoon-like, across the wide, vertical space, leaving rubble in its wake. Violence is apprehended retrospectively as a trace. As David Harris has noted, Beato 'concentrated on the ruined architecture of the North Dagu Fort as the touchstone of memory'.[48] The spectacular ruins of Beato's war photographs anticipate his subsequent pictures of the Summer Palace complex, destroyed by the Allies in mid–October 1860. Panoramas by Beato of Peking and its surrounding walls dwell on the city as an assemblage of strangely deserted architectural spaces.

Photographs of ruins – of crumbling walls, dilapidated temples, shrines, bridges, and palaces – fill the pages of the *Far East*, a magazine published from Yokohama and later Shanghai in the 1870s. Thomson's photographs of the Summer Palace reflect a similar preoccupation with ruination. As he notes of the ruined imperial complex in his album *Through China with a Camera* (1898): 'there we found a wilderness of ruin and devastation which it was piteous to behold. Marble slabs and sculptured ornaments that had graced one of the finest scenes in China now lay scattered everywhere among the debris and weeds'.[49] While Thomson's picturesque ruin photographs reflect an antiquarian interest in China's imperial history, they also suggest obsolescence, dereliction, and rupture. Ruins are 'architectural remnants which have lost their functionality and meaning'.[50] As Wu has noted, these ruins are still 'raw' and have 'not yet sunk into the depth of historical memory'.[51] The blurring of architectural thresholds between interior and exterior intimates a fundamental ambivalence, both spatial and temporal: ruins are at once valuable relics of the past, impediments to progress, and preconditions for the modern buildings that are destined to supersede them. Likewise, the camera is simultaneously an instrument of preservation and change, of construction and destruction.

As Harris notes, in many of Beato's urban photographs, 'the Chinese are largely absent and their culture is represented by the mute presence of their architecture'.[52] The ruin photography of this period is similarly depopulated. When they do appear, the Chinese are remote, spectral figures: 'they occupy a passive and incidental position, hovering at the edges, or because of lengthy exposures, they are reduced to an indistinct blur in the background'.[53] The shadowlike quality of these photographs is accentuated, too, by the 'blurred trail' left on the photographic plate by moving objects.[54] The occasional, ghost-like figures are present 'if only to provide a scale against which the ruins might be measured, or as an orientalising adjunct to the scene'.[55] In contrast, the British are often located 'at the centres of the photographs, exuding self-assurance and control'.[56] An uncanny urban environment of ruins, semi-ruins, and abandoned buildings thus becomes a graphic metaphor for China's opening up.[57] As the *Illustrated London News* asserted after the Allied victory in 1861: 'what a prospect is hereby opened up to us'.[58] Collapsed and collapsing buildings function as reminders of China's ruined economy, of its decaying culture, and of its people entrapped in the disintegrating structures of a pre-modern world. It was a view summed up by Thomson in 1875 when he wrote of 'the light of civilization' finally 'penetrating to the edges of the great Chinese continent, where the gloom of ages still broods over the cities'.[59]

Like many of his contemporaries, Griffith sought to meet the demands of an expatriate market for ruin photography and Chinese landscapes. In 1872, he undertook a photographic excursion to northern China.[60] Thomas Child mentions Griffith's arrival in Peking in mid-October and apparently, they toured the vicinity of the city together, taking photographs of the ruins of the Summer Palace.[61] In a review of Griffith's work produced during this trip, the *North China Herald* commented explicitly on his photographs of picturesque buildings in a 'state of neglect', including views of Tianjin, a city that had recently been at the centre of an anti-Christian massacre (1870).[62] The newspaper singled out Griffith's photographs of 'the ruins of the Cathedral and Orphanage and the graves of the unfortunate victims of the massacre' – a popular ruin site, which was photographed by Thomson and many others (Figure 4.3).[63]

This Western photographic interest in Chinese themes – specifically in buildings and ruins – converged with other traditions of metropolitan photography.

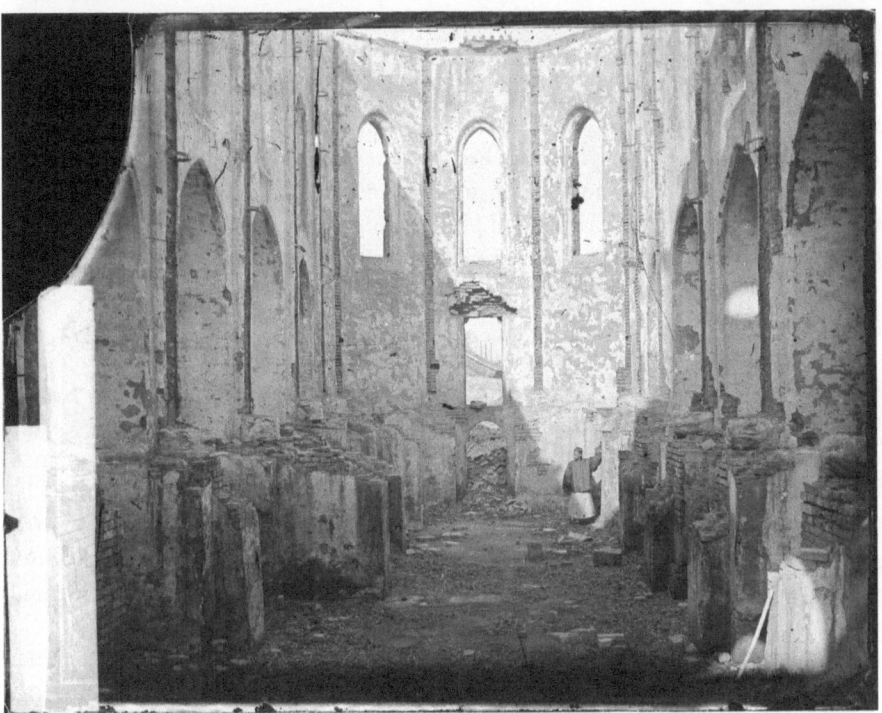

**FIGURE 4.3** John Thomson, 'Interior ruins of the Chapel of the Sisters of Charity after the Tianjin Massacre', 1871. Source: Wellcome Library, London

The interconnections between metropolitan and 'exotic' photographic worlds is perhaps best illustrated by the work of Thomson who had established a studio in Hong Kong in 1868 and travelled extensively through China, publishing the four volumes of his *Illustrations of China and Its People* between 1873 and 1874. On his return to Britain from China in 1872, Thomson sought to document the street life in London, photographing views of life on the capital's 'highways and byways', as well as 'glimpses caught here and there, at the angle of some dark alley, or in some squalid corner beyond the beat of the ordinary wayfarer'.[64] As Thomas Prasch and Nancy Armstrong have suggested, the London photographs draw on the themes and compositional techniques of the China pictures that preceded them, the one body of work offering a 'mirror image' of the other.[65]

Thomson's London photographs are, for the most part, portraits of working-class city dwellers. However, this genre of street photography overlapped with an urban slum photography that had become central to the sanitarian movement by the 1870s. Pictures of ramshackle courtyards and narrow streets transformed the sprawling industrial city into a distinct space, which the observer 'could step back from and view in much the same way he would a large object'.[66] Photography thus constituted a regimen of evidence, which was premised on impartiality and closely associated with the empirical aims of science. In this urban photography, the city tended to be pictured as a collection of vacant spaces. It was invariably imagined, as Nancy Armstrong has observed, in gothic chiaroscuro 'as a ruin or memorial to the life that had once animated it'.[67] Photography assumed an increasingly important institutional function through the 1880s and 1890s, when social reformers used it to record slum conditions and to advocate slum clearance on sanitary grounds.[68] As the Danish-American photographer and social reformer Jacob A. Riis put it in 1890, slums were 'the hot-bed of the epidemics that carry death'.[69] In turn-of-the-century exposure journalism and photography, disease was conceived first and foremost as an infrastructural, planning, and architectural problem.[70] The emphasis was consequently on photography as a means of documenting the contagious properties of buildings.[71]

The deployment of photography as part of the 'sanitarian syndrome' – and its incorporation as a crucial instrument of metropolitan government – was related to another type of photograph that celebrated the efficient infrastructure of the modern city.[72] Government offices, ports, railway stations, roads, and monumental buildings were viewed as the material foundations of the new city's commercial power. This modernisation drive involved inevitable disruptions. Urban photographs of the late nineteenth century were haunted by the prospect of the old city's impending demolition and the 'threat to place itself from the physical carving and slicing of the historical landscape and a shift in its spatial and temporal rhythms'.[73] A photography that promoted progress and advocated the destruction of urban slums conjoined with a photography that expressed nostalgia for the old city that was disappearing – a nostalgia for the about-to-be-destroyed that the cultural critic Ackbar Abbas has called, in a Hong Kong context, the '*déjà disparu*'.[74]

## Reading Griffith's *Views of the Plague*

The *Hongkong Daily Press* recorded in July 1894 that: 'Mr. D. K. Griffith has forwarded to us from his studio several photographs of an excellent series he has taken of plague scenes'.[75] The newspaper remarked how 'life-like' the photographs were, declaring that they constituted 'a permanent and faithful record' of the epidemic.[76] Among the scenes was one showing 'a party of Shropshire "lads" burning *débris* from condemned houses on a narrow filthy looking street'.[77]

In the midst of the outbreak, Griffith was offering plague photographs for sale at his studio on Duddell Street in Hong Kong's Central District. A series of thirteen photographs, described as 'Griffith's *Views of the Plague*' – with each one accompanied by a summary description – was advertised by him on 5 July. Among the series is a picture of the 'Streets and Lanes of Tai-ping-Shan', along with pictures of different stages of the anti-plague operation, including the inspection and disinfection of Chinese dwellings, and the disposal of the dead. These images were widely reproduced in the media and taken together they represent a narrative of the outbreak, conceived as interrelated 'scenes' or 'views', most of them linked by the presence of the so-called 'Whitewash Brigade'.[78]

Like other plague photographs, Griffith's images intimate the dreadfulness of the plague without showing it directly. As Helen Grace has written of the plague photographs produced by McCredie in Sydney during the outbreak there in 1900: 'the photographs do not *show* us the horror of plague but function more as a rhetorical device which evokes abjection by withholding the description of it'.[79] Griffith presents a ruinous landscape where rubbish is piled up outside the doorways of 'condemned houses'. To borrow Patrick Manson's phantasmatic term, these are 'plague-haunted houses', where the invisible germs of the 'filth disease' are imputed to fester.[80] The Chinese inhabitants are conspicuous by their absence, their nonpresence a form of ghostliness that invokes '*the sense of the presence of those who are not physically there*' (original italics).[81] The drama of Griffith's photographs lies precisely in this spectral quality; in the fact that disease is a 'phenomenological "conjuring trick"' – an 'apparition of the inapparent'.[82] What the viewer is manifestly not shown in these plague views is the plague itself. Like war or the shock of a typhoon, plague is visible only as the aftereffect of violence, in this case the violence inflicted by the colonial state's efforts to manage an invisible threat. The photographs are, in a sense, placeholders for a future meaning that will be retrospectively read into the 'view' once science has established the aetiology and transmission pathways of the plague germ.[83] In other words, the images make allowance for a retroactive interpretation. In the spring and summer of 1894, when the Hong Kong outbreak occurred, infection had yet to spread globally. It is only in hindsight that the photographs from Hong Kong can be interpreted as scenes from the beginning of the third plague pandemic. As Lynteris has noted in his discussion of epidemic photography, plague images operate simultaneously on a 'demonstrative' and 'forensic' level: while they reveal the faulty infrastructure and insalubrity that is driving disease, they also function as a type of evidentiary crime photography, capturing a 'scene' that may yield crucial evidence in future investigations.[84]

White-clad infantrymen are shown in Griffith's pictures pulling apart the potentially infected contents of the dwellings. On the one hand, the men are performing a labour. The removal of contagious debris is imagined as a form of health-production. On the other hand, the military status of these workers implicitly frames the clean-up operation as a 'campaign', with the plague inferred as a lethal enemy that requires violence to subdue. Their white apparels serve to delineate the men against the sombre backdrop of the condemned property. There is a racial symbolism to this colour-coding; the 'white' volunteers in the composition are pitted against the threat of the 'Black Death' that seeps from the native homes. This black-and-white iconography of disease echoes news reports from the 1890s that envisioned the battle against pathogens as a frontier-conflict fought between white troops and black bacterial natives.[85]

Photography is conceived as an exploratory practice. As Thomson remarked, the travel photograph was a means of enabling the distant to become newly proximate. Through photography, viewers could come 'face to face' with the objects, 'scenes and [the] people of far-off lands'.[86] Griffith's plague views are part of this 'travelling' gaze and exist as a continuum with his photographs of exploration. In 1873, Halliday Macartney, co-director of the Nanjing Arsenal, had commissioned Griffith to sail west beyond Yichang in order to secure views along the upper reaches of the Yangtze.[87] And in 1883, he had taken part in the scientific expedition of the Marchesa schooner owned and captained by C. T. Kettlewell. Reaching Hong Kong in March 1883, the boat travelled to the Philippines, visiting the Sulu Islands, British North Borneo, Batavia, Sumbawa, and New Guinea. In the subsequent book of the journey, written up by the British naturalist Francis Henry Hill Guillemard (1852–1933), Griffith provided the negatives from which 'the illustrations of tropical types and scenery [were] engraved'.[88]

The plague houses (like the ruins of war or the wreckage of a typhoon) areanti-monuments, derelict spaces that contrast to the colony's grandiose new buildings, which by the 1890s lined Queen's Road Central and the Praya. Nineteenth-century studios in Hong Kong and the treaty ports specialised in views of imposing colonial constructions, which featured on popular postcards. Like ruins, such buildings were pictured 'whole, uncropped, and often in isolation – figures or street traffic rarely appear, though a posed figure is occasionally included to give an indication of scale'.[89] A Hong Kong panorama based on a Griffith photograph, showing the colony's landmark buildings, had appeared in the *Graphic* in 1887. A caption by Griffith extolled the city's architectural transformation:

> all this is the work of less than half a century. From a barren rock, with a few
> fishing villages, Hong Kong has grown under our rule to be a most extensive

and prosperous colony, with a population of nearly a quarter of a million inhabitants.[90]

The distinction between 'English buildings' and decrepit 'Chinese buildings' reflected a moral gulf that divided colonial and native worlds. As the missionary John Macgowan remarked in 1897, Hong Kong's buildings exemplified character. He noted, for example, the insubstantial, jerry-built matsheds, shacks, and plague-ridden tenements where Chinese labourers lived. In contrast, he lauded the new offices of the Hong Kong and Shanghai Banking Corporation (HSBC), built in 1885, 'which attract the attention by the magnificence and solidity with which they have been constructed'.[91] According to Macgowan:

> the strength of the English character was never more fully manifested in the East than it is in the strong and massive houses reared in Hong-Kong. They seem as though they were intended to last a thousand years, and to defy all the effects of climate and the fierce blasts of the typhoon. Permanency is the one thought that is inscribed in unwritten language upon the structures of this town.[92]

The colony's edifying stone buildings – 'solid', 'strong', 'massive', 'permanent' – are symbolic of British commercial and military power. They are also antithetical to the flimsy native architecture, which mirrors the evanescence of its float-ing inhabitants. To borrow Macgowan's phrase, other messages are 'inscribed in unwritten language' on Chinese dwellings.[93] Photographs of these buildings recapitulate and extend the content of government reports and news articles devoted to the vexing problem of the colony's housing and specifically to the insalubrious conditions of the Chinese quarters. While the houses themselves are deemed to be badly situated and structurally defective with an 'utterly inad-equate supply of light and ventilation', they are also filled with 'dirt and rubbish' to the extent that many colonials wondered 'where the occupant can find room for himself'.[94] In a characteristic manoeuvre, Governor Des Voeux justified the European District Preservation Ordinance of 1888, which reserved part of the town for 'houses built according to European models', on the grounds that Europeans had been effectively 'pushed out' of Victoria by the unhygienic living arrangements of the Chinese.[95] Through 'a long process of natural selection', Des Voeux contended, the native population had become inured to living in closely packed houses, as opposed to Europeans, who required 'breathing space'.[96] This juxtaposition of unhealthy 'Chinese' buildings and sturdy 'English' buildings mirrors a contrast within colonial medical photography between images of the body before and after treatment – a technique that 'was widely used by medical missionaries and colonial doctors to present ocular evidence of disease, diagnosis and cure, in which the images offered a narrative about the redemptive power of Western medicine'.[97]

The floating population that inhabits these damaged local dwellings is reflective of a deeper geological instability. As the engineer and sanitarian Osbert Chadwick remarked in his 1882 *Reports on the Sanitary Condition of Hong Kong*, the ground of the colony was itself deficient; its flawed composition, which was the result of violent geological processes, led to landslides and required the construction of 'artificial ground' as a stabilising countermeasure. In Chadwick's words, 'the soil on which the city is built is derived from the decomposition of granite or other primitive rock'. Hong Kong's 'primitive' terrain is described as a 'friable mass' with uneven blocks of granite and fever-inducing water trapped 'at no great depth below the surface'.[98]

External shock could expose the true character of buildings and their occupants. If sturdy colonial edifices were designed to 'defy all the effects of climate and the fierce blasts of the typhoon', native homes were unsound and easily destroyed.[99] The colonial official and missionary Ernest Eitel noted in 1895 that Hong Kong's architecture had developed expressly as a response to the shock of typhoons. In 1841, as the colony was being established, 'a terrific typhoon' had struck, levelling the colony's hastily erected buildings: 'houses, booths and shanties were shattered and their fragments whirled through the air'.[100] 'The general impression among foreigners', Eitel declared, 'was that "the last days of Hongkong seemed to be approaching"'.[101] A similarly apocalyptic vision of post-typhoon Hong Kong is described by Mary Crawford Fraser, wife of the British diplomat Hugh Fraser, who arrived in the colony in the immediate aftermath of the 22–23 September 1874 typhoon, which left 'half of the buildings roofless ruins'. Some 2,000 persons were reported to have been killed and the atmosphere, according to Fraser, was that 'of a vast charnel house'.[102]

The devastation of the 1874 typhoon – one 'of unprecedented suddenness and power' – was captured by photographers, among them William Pryor Floyd (1830–c. 1900) and Lai Afong, the Chinese photographer whose studio Griffith had joined as an assistant in 1878.[103] News of the typhoon's destruction also made it into newspapers such as the *Illustrated London News*, which carried images of the colony's 'ruins'.[104] Eitel likened the scene to that of a war, remarking that 'the town looked as if had undergone a terrific bombardment. Thousands of houses were unroofed, hundreds of European and Chinese dwellings were in ruins'.[105] Like the photographs of war and ruin discussed above, typhoon photographs focus on the devastated city: on collapsed stone masonry, wrecked roofs, and mangled debris.

Without the plague caption as a gloss, Griffith's views of dilapidated plague houses and heaped rubble might just as well represent a post-typhoon clean-up operation, in which – as Eitel described the 1874 typhoon – the streets are impassable, obstructed by 'roof timber, window frames and mounds of soil thrown up by the bursting of drains'.[106] Natural disaster, war, and epidemic become indexical, the one invoking the other. This indexicality constructs an environmental imaginary wherein war, natural disaster, and epidemics are viewed as connected processes of ruination that provide the preconditions for rebuilding. In September 1894, the

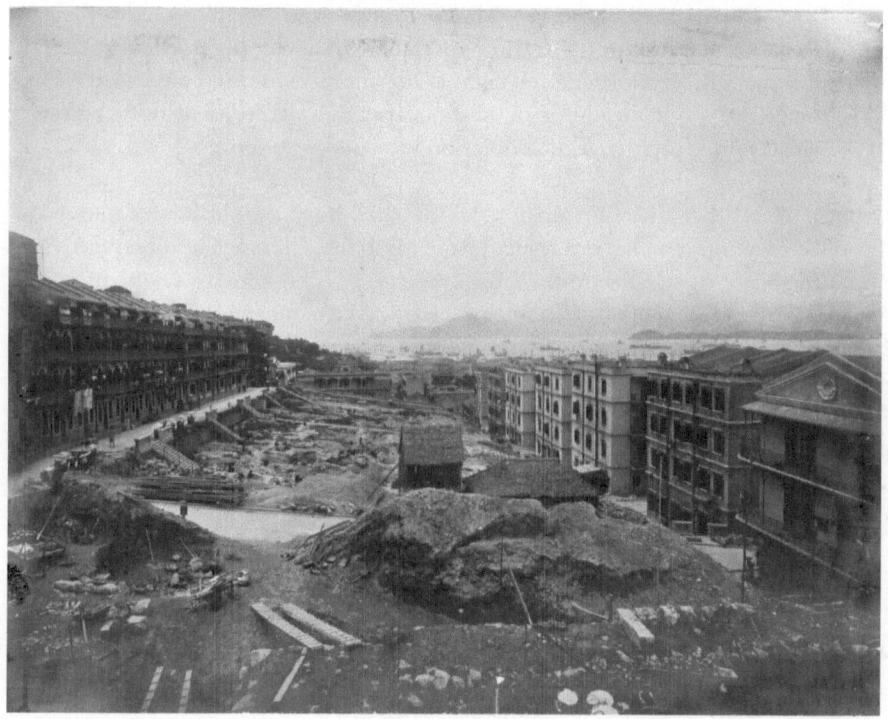

**FIGURE 4.4** 'Taipingshan. Resumed area. View of the unbuilt on portion looking westwards', after 1894. Source: National Archives, London

Taipingshan Resumption Ordinance allowed for the plague district to be 'pulled down and destroyed', in order for the area (or portions of it), to 'be laid out afresh and redrained' (Figure 4.4).[107]

As Marita Sturken has suggested, photography is crucially 'implicated in the power dynamics of memory's production'.[108] According to the *Hongkong Daily Press*, Griffith's plague views were memorials to a disaster, 'which will never be forgotten'.[109] Griffith was the 'man on the spot' – the witness and data-gatherer who jeopardised his life for the purpose of memorialising an event as it unfolded. In this sense, he resembles the amateur photographer W. E. Sharp, whose work he displayed for sale in his studio on Duddell Street. Sharp was chief engineer of the *Fatshan* who had taken a covert photograph of a grisly public execution by *lingchi* (dismemberment or 'death by a thousand cuts') in Canton. As the *Hongkong Telegraph* put it, he 'deserves a medal from the Royal Photographic Society, if there was such an institution' for tackling 'one of the most disagreeable jobs that any enthusiastic amateur could wish for':

Mr. Sharp pushed through with his camera, and, in spite of the throng, heat, the stench, and the terrible spectacle presented, obtained an excellent photograph of the gruesome sight. One more revolting could scarcely be conceived . . . to realise it in all its horror the picture itself must be seen. Mr. Griffiths [sic] has some copies on view in his studio.[110]

Griffith, like other photographers working in China, complained about local 'hostility to photographic manipulations'.[111] For the Chinese, he observed, 'the photographic image is the soul of the original'.[112] The taking of a picture was equated with the snatching of a soul and provoked fear and anger. Griffith himself had been the recipient of violence as a result of his photographic efforts: 'I have had my chair torn to pieces on the road, my coolies beaten, and my camera broken'.[113] In his plague scenes, however, we are offered an inverted spectacle of this anti-photographic Chinese violence: the central perspective of the camera converges with the viewpoint of the troops as they dismantle the Chinese dwellings. The camera is complicit in the violence it records. Here the Chinese ruins are 'back-drops' that foreground the tension between photography as an exemplary modern practice and the refractory spaces it operates in. As Arjun Appadurai puts it, such backdrops in colonial photography constitute 'sites of epistemological uncertainty about exactly what photographs seek to represent'.[114]

## Conclusion

Photographs of the third plague pandemic are too often detached from the context of their production and reception. They are presented as *de facto* evidence and 'put to work in "illustrating" arguments with little regard for the technical, percep-tual, and political work that photography can do'.[115] In contrast, this chapter has suggested that plague views from Hong Kong should be understood within the complex and uneven visual terrain of 'China' as it was being constructed at the turn of the nineteenth and twentieth centuries.[116]

Understanding the history of the multiple generic threads that constitute epi-demic photography is important for a number of reasons. First, it provides a means of glimpsing how those caught up in outbreak episodes make sense of them. In this way, it may also help us to think afresh about the evolution of the 'epidemic' as an epidemiological category, suggesting an overlap with other species of natural disaster and anthropogenic violence, including typhoons and war. Indeed, a sketch based on a Griffith photograph of the 'Whitewash Brigade' appeared in the *Graphic* on 29 December, alongside an illustration showing the clearing of wreckage caused by a calamitous earthquake in Constantinople and Greece.[117] Under the heading 'Calamities and Accidents', the newspaper declared: 'the debit side in the world's balance-sheet for 1894 has a heavy item under the "calamity" rubric'.[118] The edito-rial provided an overview of disparate catastrophes that had taken place across the world in 1894, causing panic and loss of life. Beginning with an account of the earthquake, the plague in Hong Kong was evoked in relation to disastrous floods, cyclones, and forest fires.[119]

Second, studying a photograph as a 'biographical object' – that is, as an object with its own history rather than as an illustration of an historical event – restores specificity to the image and reminds us that photographs of the third plague pandemic need to be viewed as contextually-determined visual documents.[120] Too often, colonial photography is identified as an imperial phenomenon as if there were no substantive difference between works produced by photographers, say, in Hong Kong, Bombay, or Burma. Similarity of technique and style, and the recurrence of motifs across colonial sites – images of tenements, street views, government inspections, and suchlike – can be misleading. Plague photographs from China drew their force from an inferred relation to other non-plague images of Chinese places and people. Recognising the particularities of photographic encounters – their dependency on context – may help to decentre imperial photography, pushing back against global histories that lose sight of difference and diversity. As Wu Hung has aptly observed, a nineteenth-century photograph was 'not only an image of historical figures or buildings but also a visual construct made at a specific moment by an individual photographer or a commercial studio for particular purposes'.[121]

Third, examining the multiple prehistories of the epidemic photograph encourages us to reassess prevailing assumptions about the interrelationship between cities, late nineteenth-century sanitary science, and disease. Plague photography drew on a tradition of metropolitan slum-clearance photography. However, the degree to which this sanitarian dimension was integrated into other traditions of travel and reportage reminds us of the continuities that are often overlooked in accounts of hygienic modernity. Tracking the plague through the manifold visual representations of ruination that coexisted in the 1890s reveals the imperial album as an uneasy accommodation of scales. If visual fragments could assemble into a narrative – the third plague pandemic – this narrative was only illusory; for in the process of viewing plague, the plague vanished across the multiple sites of its representation.

During the 2003 SARS outbreak in Hong Kong, the plagued city was depicted in the global media as a ruined city: desolate streets, empty tower blocks, lone masked passengers on the MTR, the ghostly fluorescence of abandoned restaurants. Disseminated online, these twenty-first-century plague views were anticipatory, signalling the pandemic to come. Yet this emphasis on immanence – on 'pandemic prophecy' as it has been called – obscures the historicity of the visual templates that structure how the future is imagined.[122] As this chapter has suggested, epidemic photography as it developed in China at the turn of the nineteenth and twentieth centuries drew on antecedents: on images of ruin, war, and natural disaster. Tracing the ways in which 'plague scenes' have been historically assembled can provide new understanding of the inherited templates that structure contemporary epidemic photography. It may also furnish an effective means of challenging the assumed connections between certain locales and the 'wilderness of ruin' that enables disease's emergence.

## Notes

1  On the landscape of influenza in southern China, see Wallace *et al.*, 'Epidemiology'; on SARS, as the first 'plague' of the twenty-first century, see Abraham, *Twenty-First Century Plague.*
2  Wald, *Contagious*, 6–8; Lynteris, 'Prophetic Faculty', 121–123.
3  Serlin, 'Introduction', xiv; on the transience of 'non-places' see Augé, *Non-Places.*
4  Peckham, *Epidemics*, 296. On the prehistory of this global reversal, see Peckham, 'Infective Economies', 212.
5  Wald, *Contagious*, 7.
6  Ali and Keil, 'Introduction', 1.
7  See, for example, Tormey, *Cities*; Tucker, *Nature*; Serlin, 'Introduction'; Sheehan, *Doctored*; Lynteris and Prince, 'Anthropology'.
8  Lynteris, 'Prophetic Faculty', where he develops the notion of 'epidemic photography', 123. The special issue of the journal *Visual Anthropology* 29, 2 (2016) provides a useful overview of the theoretical issues at stake in the interpretation of epidemic photographs.
9  See Lynteris, 'Prophetic Faculty'.
10  For a general account of the third plague pandemic, see Echenberg, *Plague.*
11  Worswick, 'Photography', 143.
12  Legge, *Guide*, 39.
13  See *Plague Visitation, Bombay, 1896–1897*, India Office, British Library, 311/1–2. On McCredie, see Grace, 'New Journal'.
14  Des Voeux, 'Report', 300. To date, there is no comprehensive history of photography in Hong Kong that examines its diverse uses by the state. Photographs of registered brothel prostitutes were made mandatory under Section 33 of the Women's and Girls' Protection Ordinance, 1890; see 'Government Notification No. 122', *Hongkong Government Gazette* (hereafter *HGG*) (21 March 1891), 194–195; see also, 'Tender for Photographing Prisoners of Victoria Goal' ('Government Notification No. 115'), *HGG* (25 May 1872), 281.
15  Quoted in Munn, 'Hong Kong', 391–392.
16  Peckham, 'Matshed Laboratory', 145.
17  James, 'Report', 337. Wittenberg's photographic views of Meizhou are available at the University of Southern California's 'International Mission Photography' (IMP) archive: http://digitallibrary.usc.edu/.
18  Pinney, 'Introduction', 3–4.
19  David Arnold has convincingly argued that the Indian plague archive should be viewed 'within a longer lineage of mass representation' extending from depictions of 'famine sufferers' in the 1870s to riots in the 1920s and images of partition in 1947; Arnold, 'India'.
20  See Hevia, 'Photographic Complex'.
21  On the 'visual archive of ruination', see Hell and Schönle, 'Introduction', 1.
22  The term 'evidentiary crescendo' is borrowed from Pinney, 'Introduction', 1.
23  On 'media templates' in relation to 'framing', see Kitzinger, 'Media', 75–77.
24  Wald, *Contagious*; Rosenberg, 'What Is an Epidemic?', 279, 280–281.
25  Hong Kong was formally constituted as a crown colony in June 1843.
26  'Report on the Census of the Colony for 1901', *Hongkong Sessional Papers for 1901* (hereafter *HSP*), Table 1, 9.
27  Sinn, 'Lesson'.
28  Lau, *Picturing*, 3.

29  'Actualités: la Chine étant ouverte attire immédiatement à Pekin tous les photographes, qui se mettent en mesure de saisir sa majesté impériale dès sa sortie du palais', *Le charivari* (25 October 1858), 564.

30  On the growing Western ambivalence to China and Chinese 'things' in the second half of the nineteenth century, see Peckham, 'Hong Kong Junk'.

31  Harris, *Of Battle*; Thiriez, *Barbarian Lens*.

32  Ricalton, *China*.

33  For an (albeit incomplete) overview of Griffith's life, see Bennett, *History*, 268–279. Griffith died on 2 January 1897 in the Government Civil Hospital in Hong Kong and was buried in Happy Valley on 4 January. A notice in the *Hongkong Telegraph* mentions a niece and a married sister in the East; see *Hongkong Telegraph* (4 January 1897), 2; also *North China Herald* (15 January 1897), 9.

34  According to the 1861 census, Griffith was then living as a boarder in a house on Albany Street in Regent's Park, London, and his occupation is given as 'artist'. An advertisement for 'photographic instruction' by Griffith appeared in the *Worcester Chronicle* (27 April 1864). Later in the 1860s, he was working in Norwich and is listed in the Norfolk Register of Electors. From July 1868, Griffith was taking out advertisements in the Norfolk press for 'artistic photographs'; see, for example, the advertisement in the *Norfolk News* (5 September 1868). *Carte de visite* photographs produced by Griffith during this period are contained in the 'Carte de visite photographs album of families of Norfolk County, England, between 1865 and 1910' deposited at the University of California, Los Angeles, Special Collections, Charles E. Young Research Library, 94/168.

35  See the notice announcing that Griffith has joined Lai Afong's studio in the *China Mail* (11 July 1878), 2; see also the advertisement for Griffith's studio in the *China Mail* (24 May 1884), 2; on Griffith's photographs for the 1886 exhibition, see *China Mail* (21 November 1885), 2. Between 1883–1885, Griffith is also listed as a soda water manufacturer; see the advertisement for 'D. K. Griffith & Co. Manufacturers of the London Aerated Waters and General Agents. Established for the Manufacture of Superior Aerated Drinks', which appeared in Eastlake, *Guide*.

36  'The Plague at Hong-Kong', *Illustrated London News* (28 July 1894), 100; *Graphic* (4 August 1894), 120.

37  The phrase 'incontestable pictorial evidence' is taken from the preface in Thomson's *Through China*, v.

38  Echenberg, *Plague*, 30, 42.

39  Barthes, *Camera*, 19. A photograph showing a scene from the outbreak of the plague in Honolulu, Hawaii, in 1899, is reproduced on the front of Echenberg's book; for a discussion of this image and the implications of disconnecting a photograph from its 'archival locality', see Poleykett, Evans, and Engelmann, 'Fragments'.

40  Prince, 'Diseased Body', 162, 165. On the 'social biography' of the photograph as material object in the colonial archive, see Edwards, 'Material Beings', 68; Edwards and Hart, 'Mixed Box'.

41  Tagg, *Burden*, 2; in particular, note his comment: 'Photographs are never "evidence" of history; they are themselves the historical', 65.

42  Hevia, 'Photography Complex', 81.

43  Wu, 'Introduction', 12–15. For an insightful study of the ways in which ruins have been interpellated back into Chinese art and visual culture, see Hung, *Story*.

44  Sontag, *Regarding the Pain*, 45–46.

45  Thomson, *Through Cyprus*, I, vi. See also Sterling who discusses Thomson's Cypriot ruins in 'Spectral Anatomies'.

46  Wu, 'Ruins', 60. On the relationship between photography and Orientalism, generally, see the contributions in Behdad and Gartlan, *Photography's Orientalism*.

47  On the performative qualities of documentary photography, see Edwards, *Raw Histories*.

48  Harris, *Of Battle*, 31.

49 Thomson, *Through China*, 263.
50 Hell and Schönle, 'Introduction', 6.
51 Wu, *Ruins*, 60, where the term 'ashes' is proposed to designate these ruins in order 'to distinguish them from those aestheticised ruin images in classical poems'; on documentary photography and 'raw history', see Edwards, *Raw Histories*.
52 Harris, *Of Battle*, 27.
53 *Ibid.*
54 Cécile Léon Art Projects, *First Photographs*, 93.
55 Sterling, 'Spectral Anatomies'.
56 Harris, *Of Battle*, 27.
57 On the German photographer Ernst Ohlmer, see Warren, 'Romanticising'.
58 Chang, *Britain's Chinese Eye*, 141.
59 Thomson, *Straits*, vi.
60 Griffith, 'A Rolling Stone's Visit'.
61 Bennett, *History*, 270, 287. However, as yet I have found no mention by Griffith of his association with Child.
62 'Summary of News', *North China Herald* (19 December 1872), 527.
63 *Ibid.*
64 'Preface', in: Thomson and Smith, *Street Life*.
65 Prasch, 'Mirror Images'; Armstrong, *Fiction*, 104–106. See also Chang, *Britain's Chinese Eye*, 152–163.
66 Armstrong, 'City Things', 106.
67 *Ibid.*, 108–109.
68 Tagg, *Burden*, 129.
69 Riis, *How the Other Half Lives*, 3; Tagg, *Burden*, 196.
70 On 'exposure' photography during this period, see Yochelson and Czitrom, *Rediscovering*.
71 See Peckham, 'Pathological Properties', 56–57, where the work of Eugène Atget is discussed.
72 Swanson, 'Sanitation Syndrome'.
73 Edwards, *Camera*, 135.
74 Abbas, *Hong Kong*, 16.
75 'The Plague', *Hongkong Daily Press* (6 July 1894), 2.
76 *Ibid.*
77 *Ibid.*
78 On which, see Platt, Jones, and Platt, *Whitewash Brigade*.
79 Grace, 'New Journal', 76.
80 Manson, *Tropical Diseases*, 151; 'Governor's Despatch on the Incipience and Progress of the Plague in the Colony During 1896' (6 May 1896), *HSP*, 449–455 (452).
81 Bell, 'Ghosts', 813; see also Sterling, 'Spectral Anatomies'.
82 These terms are borrowed from Derrida, *Specters*, 125–176.
83 A description of Griffith's plague photographs appeared in the same newspaper article that described the view of the plague bacilli as seen through Yersin's microscope; see 'The Plague', *Hongkong Daily Press* (6 July 1894), 2. Illustrative plates of the bacilli accompanied Yersin's 1894 article, 'Peste bubonique'.
84 Lynteris, 'Prophetic Faculty', 125–126.
85 Tucker, *Nature*, 188–191.
86 Thomson, *Through China*, vii. On the relationship between laboratory science, exploration, and photography, see Peckham, 'Matshed Laboratory', 145.
87 See Griffith's letter to Dr Macartney (17 July 1873) reproduced in Boulger, *Life*, 212–213. Cited in Bickers, 'Lives', 19.
88 Guillemard, *Cruise*, 189. On the cruise, see [Moses & Co] *Straits Times* (21 January 1884), 3; *Ibid.* (20 September 1887), 2.
89 Wue, 'Picturing Hong Kong', 41.
90 'The City of Victoria, Hongkong', *Graphic* (26 February 1887), 211; the engraving based on Griffith's photograph and entitled 'Panorama of the Town of Victoria, Hongkong' appears on 224–225.

91  Macgowan, *Pictures*, 240.
92  *Ibid.*, 240–241.
93  *Ibid.*, 241.
94  'Governor's Despatch on the Incipience and Progress of the Plague in the Colony During 1896' (6 May 1896), *HSP*, 449–455; on the rubbish that cluttered Chinese houses, see Peckham, 'Hong Kong Junk'.
95  Des Voeux, 'Report', 293.
96  *Ibid.*
97  Prince, 'Diseased Body', 161.
98  Chadwick, *Mr. Chadwick's Reports*, 7.
99  Macgowan, *Pictures*, 241.
100  Eitel, *Europe*, 175.
101  *Ibid.*, 175–176.
102  Fraser, *Diplomatist's Wife*, II, 96.
103  Eitel, *Europe*, 514.
104  'The Late Typhoon at Hong-Kong: H. M. Gun-Boat Flamer Amidst the Ruins of the Boat-House and Swimming-Bath', *Illustrated London News* (21 November 1874), 196.
105  Eitel, *Europe*, 514.
106  *Ibid.*
107  'Government Notification No. 364', *HGG* (29 September 1894), 843–856 (845).
108  Sturken, *Tangled Memories*, 10.
109  'The Plague', *Hongkong Daily Press* (6 July 1894), 2.
110  'Local and General', *Hongkong Telegraph* (17 June 1890), 2. The Royal Photographic Society was in fact founded in 1894.
111  Griffith, 'A Celestial Studio', 260.
112  *Ibid.*
113  *Ibid.*
114  Appadurai, 'Colonial Backdrop', 4.
115  Poleykett, Evans, and Engelmann, 'Fragments'.
116  Wu, 'Introduction', 2.
117  'Calamities and Accidents', *Graphic* (19 December 1894), 12.
118  *Ibid.*
119  *Ibid.*
120  Prince, 'Diseased Body', 162.
121  Wu, 'Introduction', 1; see also the essays collected in Sheehan, *Photography*.
122  Carduff, *Pandemic*; Lynteris, 'Prophetic Faculty'.

# References

Abbas, Ackbar, *Hong Kong: Culture and the Politics of Disappearance* (Hong Kong: Hong Kong University Press, 1997).

Abraham, Thomas, *Twenty-First Century Plague: The Story of SARS* (Hong Kong: Hong Kong University Press, 2004).

Ali, Syed Harris and Roger Keil, 'Introduction: Networked Disease', in: S. Harris Ali and Roger Keil (eds.), *Networked Disease: Emerging Infections in the Global City* (Malden: Blackwell, 2008), 1–8.

Appadurai, Arjun, 'The Colonial Backdrop', *Afterimage*, 24, 5 (1997), 4–7.

Armstrong, Nancy, 'City Things: Photography and the Urbanization Process', in: Diana Fuss (ed.), *Human, All Too Human* (New York and London: Routledge, 1996), 93–100.

Armstrong, Nancy, *Fiction in the Age of Photography: The Legacy of British Realism* (Cambridge, MA: Harvard University Press, 1999).

Arnold, David, 'India and the Third Plague Pandemic', unpublished lecture, Wolfson College, University of Cambridge, 22 May 2014.

Augé, Marc, *Non-Places: Introduction to an Anthropology of Supermodernity*, John Howe (trans.) (London and New York: Verso, 1995).

Barthes, Roland, *Camera Lucida*, Richard Howard (trans.) (New York: Noonday Press, 1981).

Behdad, Ali and Luke Gartlan (eds.), *Photography's Orientalism: New Essays on Colonial Representation* (Los Angeles: Getty Research Institute, 2013).

Bell, Michael Mayerfeld, 'The Ghosts of Place', *Theory and Society*, 26, 6 (1997), 813–836.

Bennett, Terry, *History of Photography in China: Western Photographers, 1861–1879* (London: Quaritch, 2010).

Bickers, Robert, 'Lives & Deaths of Photographs in Early Treaty Port China', in: Henriot, Christian and Wen-hsin Yeh (eds.), *Visualising China, 1845–1965* (Leiden and Boston: Brill, 2013), 3–38.

Boulger, Demetrius C., *The Life of Sir Halliday Macartney* (London: Bodley Head, 1908).

Caduff, Carlo, *The Pandemic Perhaps: Dramatic Events in a Public Culture of Danger* (Berkeley: University of California Press, 2015).

Cécile Léon Art Projects, *First Photographs of Hong Kong, 1858–1875* (Oxford: Oxford University Press, 2010).

Chadwick, Osbert, *Mr. Chadwick's Reports on the Sanitary Condition of Hong Kong; With Appendices and Plans* (London: Colonial Office, 1882).

Chang, Elizabeth Hope, *Britain's Chinese Eye: Literature, Empire, and Aesthetics in Nineteenth-Century Britain* (Stanford, CA: Stanford University Press, 2010).

Derrida, Jacques, *Specters of Marx: The State of the Debt, the Work of Mourning, and the New International*, Peggy Kamuf (trans.) (New York and London: Routledge, 1994).

Des Voeux, Sir G. William, 'Report on the Condition and Prospects of Hongkong' (31 October), *Hongkong Sessional Papers for 1889* (1889), 289–304.

Eastlake, F. Warrington, *A Guide to Hongkong* (Hong Kong: W. Brewer, Bookseller, 1883).

Echenberg, Myron, *Plague Ports: The Global Urban Impact of Bubonic Plague, 1894–1901* (New York: New York University Press, 2007).

Edwards, Elizabeth, 'Material Beings: Objecthood and Ethnographic Photographs', *Visual Studies*, 17, 1 (2002), 67–75.

Edwards, Elizabeth, *Raw Histories: Photographs, Anthropology and Museums* (Oxford: Berg, 2001).

Edwards, Elizabeth, *The Camera as Historian: Amateur Photographers and Historical Imagination, 1885–1918* (Durham, NC: Duke University Press, 2012).

Edwards, Elizabeth and Janice Hart, 'Mixed Box: The Cultural Biography of a Box of 'Ethnographic' Photographs', in: Elizabeth Edwards and Janice Hart (eds.), *Photographs, Objects, Histories: On the Materiality of Images* (New York and London: Routledge, 2004), 47–61.

Eitel, Ernest, *Europe in China: The History of Hongkong from the Beginning to the Year 1882* (Hong Kong: Kelly and Walsh, 1895).

Fraser, Mrs. Hugh, *A Diplomatist's Wife in Many Lands* (New York: Dodd, Mead, and Company, 1910).

Guillemard, F. H. H., *The Cruise of the Marchesa to Kamschatka & New Guinea: With Notices of Formosa, Liu-Kiu, and Various Islands of the Malay Archipelago* (London: John Murray, 1889 [1886]).

Grace, Helen, 'A New Journal of the Plague Year', *Cultural Studies*, 1, 1 (1987), 75–91.

Griffith, D. K., 'A Celestial Studio', *Photographic News*, 19 (1875), 259–261.

Griffith, D. K., 'A Rolling Stone's Visit to Pekin', *Photographic News* (28 May 1875), 512–513, 520–525.

Harris, David, *Of Battle and Beauty: Felice Beato's Photographs of China* (Santa Barbara, CA: Santa Barbara Museum of Art, 1999).

Hell, Julia and Andreas Schönle, 'Introduction', in: Julia Hell and Andreas Schönle (eds.), *Ruins of Modernity* (Durham, NC: Duke University Press, 2010), 1–14.

Hevia, James, 'The Photography Complex: Exposing Boxer Era China (1900–1901), Making Civilization', in: Rosalind C. Morris (ed.), *Photographies East: The Camera and Its Histories in East and Southeast Asia* (Durham, NC: Duke University Press, 2009), 79–119.

James, H. E. R., 'A Report on the Epidemic of Bubonic Plague, which Occurred in Hong Kong in the Months of May, June, and July, 1894, with Six Diagrams', *Army Medical Department Report for the Year 1893 with Appendix, Vol. 35* (London: Her Majesty's Stationery Office, 1895), 330–356.

Kitzinger, Jenny, 'Media Templates: Patterns of Association and the (Re)Construction of Meaning over Time', *Media, Culture & Society*, 22, 1 (2000), 61–84.

Lau, Grace, *Picturing the Chinese: Early Western Photographs and Postcards of China* (Hong Kong: Joint Publishing, 2008).

Legge, William, *A Guide to Hongkong with Some Remarks Upon Macao and Canton* (Hong Kong: Walter W. Brewer, 1893).

Lynteris, Christos, 'The Prophetic Faculty of Epidemic Photography: Chinese Wet Markets and the Imagination of the Next Pandemic', *Visual Anthropology*, 29, 2 (2016), 118–132.

Lynteris, Christos and Ruth J. Prince, 'Anthropology and Medical Photography: Ethnographic, Critical and Comparative Perspectives', *Visual Anthropology*, 29, 2 (2016), 107–117.

Macgowan, John, *Pictures of Southern China* (London: Religious Tract Society, 1897).

Manson, Patrick, *Tropical Diseases: A Manual of the Diseases of Warm Climates* (London: Cassell, 1898).

Munn, Christopher, 'Hong Kong, 1841–1870', in: Douglas Hay and Paul Craven (eds.), *Masters, Servants, and Magistrates in Britain and the Empire, 1562–1955* (Chapel Hill: University of North Carolina Press, 2004), 365–401.

Peckham, Robert, *Epidemics in Modern Asia* (Cambridge, UK: Cambridge University Press, 2016).

Peckham, Robert, 'Hong Kong Junk: Plague and the Economy of Chinese Things', *Bulletin of the History of Medicine*, 90, 1 (2016), 32–60.

Peckham, Robert, 'Infective Economies: Empire, Panic and the Business of Disease', *Journal of Imperial and Commonwealth History*, 41, 2 (2013), 211–237.

Peckham, Robert, 'Matshed Laboratory: Colonies, Cultures, and Bacteriology', in: Robert Peckham and David M. Pomfret (eds.), *Imperial Contagions: Medicine, Hygiene, and Cultures of Planning in* Asia (Hong Kong: Hong Kong University Press, 2013), 123–147.

Peckham, Robert, 'Pathological Properties: Scenes of Crime, Sites of Infection', in: Robert Peckham (ed.), *Disease and Crime: A History of Social Pathologies and the New Politics of Health* (New York: Routledge, 2014), 56–78.

Pinney, Christopher, 'Introduction: "How the Other Half . . ."', in: Christopher Pinney and Nicolas Peterson (eds.), *Photography's Other Histories* (Durham, NC: Duke University Press, 2003), 1–14.

Platt, Jerome J., Maurice E. Jones, and Arleen Kay Platt, *The Whitewash Brigade: The Hong Kong Plague, 1894* (London: Dix Noonan Webb, 1998).

Poleykett, Branwyn, Nicholas H. A. Evans, and Lukas Engelmann, 'Fragments of Plague', *Limn* 6 (March 2016): http://limn.it/fragments-of-plague/.

Prasch, Thomas, 'Mirror Images: John Thomson's Photographs of East Asia', in: Douglas Kerr and Julia Kuehn (eds.), *A Century of Travels in China: Critical Essays on Travel Writing from the 1840s to the 1940s* (Hong Kong: Hong Kong University Press, 2007), 53–62.

Prince, Ruth J., 'The Diseased Body and the Global Subject: The Circulation and Consumption of an Iconic AIDS Photograph in East Africa', *Visual Anthropology*, 29, 2 (2016), 159–186.

Ricalton, James, *China Through the Stereoscope: A Journey Through the Dragon Empire at the Time of the Boxer Uprising* (New York and London: Underwood & Underwood, 1901).

Riis, Jacob A., *How the Other Half Lives: Studies among the Tenements of New York* (New York: Charles Scribner's Sons, 1890).

Rosenberg, Charles E., 'What Is an Epidemic? AIDS in Historical Perspective', in: Charles E. Rosenberg, *Explaining Epidemics and Other Studies in the History of Medicine* (Cambridge, UK: Cambridge University Press, 1992), 278–292.

Sterling, Colin, 'Spectral Anatomies: Heritage Hauntology and the "Ghosts" of Varosha', *Present Pasts: Research Papers* (February 2014): doi:10.5334/pp.57.

Serlin, David, 'Introduction: Toward a Visual Culture of Public Health: From Broadside to YouTube', in: David Serlin (ed.), *Imagining Illness: Public Health and Visual Culture* (Minneapolis: University of Minnesota Press, 2010), xi–xxxvii.

Sheehan, Tanya, *Doctored: The Medicine of Photography in Nineteenth-Century America* (University Park: Pennsylvania State University Press, 2011).

Sheehan, Tanya, (ed.), *Photography, History, Difference* (Hanover, NH: Dartmouth College Press, 2014).

Sinn, Elizabeth, 'Lesson in Openness: Creating a Space of Flow in Hong Kong', in: Helen F. Siu and Agnes S. Ku (eds.), *Hong Kong Mobile: Making a Global Population* (Hong Kong: Hong Kong University Press, 2008), 13–43.

Sontag, Susan, *Regarding the Pain of Others* (London: Hamish Hamilton, 2003).

Swanson, Maynard W., 'The Sanitation Syndrome: Bubonic Plague and Urban Native Policy in the Cape Colony, 1900–1909', *Journal of African History*, 18, 3 (1977), 387–410.

Sturken, Marita, *Tangled Memories: The Vietnam War, the Aids Epidemic, and the Politics of Remembering* (Berkeley: University of California Press, 1997).

Tagg, John, *The Burden of Representation: Essays on Photographies and Histories* (Basingstoke: Macmillan, 1988).

Thiriez, Régine, *Barbarian Lens: Western Photographers of the Qianlong Emperor's European Palaces* (Amsterdam: Gordon Breach, 1998).

Thomson, John, *Through China with a Camera* (London: A. Constable & Co., 1898).

Thomson, John, *Through Cyprus with the Camera in the Autumn of 1878*, 2 Vols. (London: Sampson, Low, Marston, Searle, & Rivington, 1879).

Thomson, John, *The Straits of Malacca, Indo-China, and China or, Ten Years' Travels, Adventures, and Residence Abroad* (London: Sampson Low, Marston, Low, & Searle, 1875).

Thomson, John and Adolphe Smith, *Street Life in London* (London: Sampson Low, Marston, Searle, & Rivington, 1877).

Tormey, Jane, *Cities and Photography* (Abingdon and New York: Routledge, 2013).

Tucker, Jennifer, *Nature Exposed: Photography as Eyewitness in Victorian Science* (Baltimore, MD: Johns Hopkins University Press, 2005).

Wald, Priscilla, *Contagious: Cultures, Carriers, and the Outbreak Narrative* (Durham, NC: Duke University Press, 2008).

Wallace, Robert G., Luke Bergmann, Lenny Hogerwerf, and Marius Gilbert, 'Are Influenzas in Southern China Byproducts of the Region's Globalising Historical Present?', in: Tamara Giles-Vernick and Susan Craddock, with Jennifer Gunn (eds.), *Influenza and Public Health: Learning from Past Pandemics* (London and Washington, DC: Earthscan, 2010), 101–144.

Warren, Maureen, 'Romanticising the Uncanny: Ernst Ohlmer's 1873 Photographs of the European-style Palaces of the Yuanmingyuan', in: Micheline Nilsen (ed.), *Nineteenth-Century*

*Photographs and Architecture: Documenting History, Charting Progress, and Exploring the World* (Farnham: Ashgate, 2013), 233–250.

Worswick, Clark, 'Photography in Imperial China', in: Clark Worswick and Jonathan Spence (eds.), *Imperial China: Photographs, 1850–1912* (New York: Pennwick/Crown, 1978), 134–149.

Wu, Hung, *A Story of Ruins: Presence and Absence in Chinese Art and Visual Culture* (London: Reaktion, 2012).

Wu, Hung, 'Introduction: Reading Early Photographs of China', in: Jeffrey W. Cody and Frances Terpak (eds.), *Brush & Shutter: Early Photography in China* (Los Angeles: Getty Research Institute, 2011), 1–32.

Wu, Hung, 'Ruins, Fragmentation, and the Chinese Modern/Postmodern', in: Gao Minglu (ed.), *Inside/Out: New Chinese Art* (Berkeley: University of California Press, 2013), 59–66.

Wue, Roberta, 'Picturing Hong Kong: Photography through Practice and Function', in: Roberta Wue (ed.), *Picturing Hong Kong: Photography, 1855–1910* (New York: Asia Society Galleries, 1997), 17–47.

Yersin, Alexandre, 'La peste bubonique à Hong-Kong', *Annales de l'Institut Pasteur*, 8 (1894), 662–667.

Yochelson, Bonnie and Daniel Czitrom, *Rediscovering Jacob Riis: Exposure Journalism and Photography in Turn-of-the-Century New York* (New York: New Press, 2007).

# 5

# THE DISEASE MAP AND THE CITY

Desire and imitation in the Bombay plague, 1896–1914[1]

*Nicholas H. A. Evans*

This chapter examines colonial attempts to map and visualise plague in British India, 1896–1914. It asks how mapping might have fascinated those seeking certainty in the interpretation of a disease, and it explores how colonial doctors tried to capture the power of maps in their own writing.

By the end of the nineteenth century, mapping was a well-established investigatory technique in epidemiology. Maps had been used extensively in the investigation of yellow fever in late eighteenth-century North America, and in the nineteenth century, they were important tools in the struggle to comprehend the global spread of a number of diseases, in particular cholera.[2] For many medical historians, however, these epidemiological maps are more than just representations of disease. The historian Tom Koch, for example, has shown that from the late early modern period onwards, mapping has been a crucial technique through which diseases have been made visible out of isolated local phenomena. For Koch, maps are instruments through which theories and arguments about the nature of disease have been articulated.[3] Mapping connects lived experience with investigations carried out under theoretical assumptions so as to transform disparate phenomena into something that can be known as disease. Illustrating this, Koch shows how during the nineteenth century, mapping enabled up to four quite separate choleras to be debated and argued, and, in doing so, allowed overwhelming quantities of data to be synthesised as arguments.[4] He thus shows that by the late nineteenth century, maps were essential tools through which hypotheses about disease could be articulated. Maps were crucial to scientific processes through which disparate phenomena could be argued to belong to broader events such as epidemics and pandemics, and they were central to the construction of arguments through which certainties about those disease-events could be formulated.

Beyond the study of disease, the ability of maps to produce incontestable knowledge about territories has been a continuous source of fascination for scholars of cartography.Since at least the nineteenth century, cartographers have often laid claim to neutral scientific objectivity: maps are seen as representations of the world as it really is. In the last few decades, however, a number of scholars have questioned such claims, in order to show how the power of the map to produce certainty can operate through a façade of neutral science. Brian Harley, for example, famously argued that maps might be as much images of social order as they are objective measurements of the world.[5] In this tradition of analysis, the most thorough work on cartography in colonial India is Matthew Edney's *Mapping an Empire*, which explores an ever-present tension between a cartographic ideal and actual mapping practices. While nineteenth-century surveys of British India were frequently chaotic, such anarchy could be hidden beneath a cartographic archive that sustained a myth of order, and in this way, 'the British created a geographical *myth* of an empire comprising known or knowable territory'.[6] This approach challenges any reading of cartography as a neutral science. Cartography's claims to objective representation are seen to cloak a sometimes imitative relation to reality, in which maps project themselves as objective technologies, but in so doing can mesmerise us with their mimetic power.[7] Unifying this literature is a concern to understand how maps produce a sense of their own certainty. Maps can erase complexities, and produce a fictive sense of seeing all and thus knowing all. Matthew Edney, in particular, shows that by the late nineteenth century, mapping was valued as a technique across scientific and political realms precisely because of its ability to create a certain and known image in the face of otherwise incomprehensible complexity.

This chapter asks what that sense of certainty might have meant for colonial doctors who utilised mapping as a technique to understand a plague epidemic in Bombay in the late nineteenth and early twentieth centuries. I ask how the capacity of disease maps to assert, to reason, to clarify, and to argue had, by the very end of the nineteenth century, become a part of their mythology. The plague outbreak in India created a situation of far-reaching uncertainty for the colonial administration: the mysterious aetiology of the disease pushed doctors to the limits of their own medical understanding, while also revealing the colonial state's inability to know its racial and social other.[8] In such a setting, the technology of mapping, which was understood to make arguments in a cogent fashion, could offer a certainty that was much desired.

In probing the link between desire and certainty, this chapter thus aims to contribute to our understanding of the 'mimetic powers' of maps.[9] Previous analyses of this, building upon the work of Brian Harley, have tended to focus upon cartography's seductive promise to accurately mimic 'reality' through technical skill.[10] In this chapter, I explore a further layer of mimicry, namely, the way in which cartography's promises could be mirrored and reflected *within* practices of mapping. This, in turn, can help us to understand the place of mimetic thinking within European colonialism. The anthropologist Michael Taussig has described how European colonial thought associated mimesis (an attempt to capture the power of the other through imitation) with its 'savage' other.[11] Europeans saw themselves as uniquely creative and original, while the 'primitive' subjects of their colonial expansion were seen to be innately imitative. Across the colonial world, much imperial ideology thus rested upon a narrative that dignified European scientific modernity as a break from primitive forms of mimetic reasoning. The texts and maps that I will discuss in this chapter were contemporary with James Frazer's *Golden Bough*, the early anthropological treatise which – in a broader public sphere – most clearly articulated the separation of European thought from its past as an evolution of thought on causation: if Europeans had science, their savage other had sympathetic magic, based upon a mimetic and imitative logic.[12] The modern European, in other words, was understood to have evolved beyond imitation with the discovery of reason and science. Taussig nonetheless argued that Europeans were not immune to their own mimetic excesses, and they frequently mimicked the other, often acting out the savagery that they imputed to the other.[13]

The maps explored in this chapter can further help to deconstruct colonial claims to rationality, which were based upon a hierarchical logic in which the primitive was to the modern as mimesis was to science. I will ask what might be learnt by viewing colonial disease mapping as a genre that imitated itself in a search for certain knowledge. In so doing, I will argue that some disease maps should thus be read not just as panoptic claims to know the colonial city, but also as spaces of desire in which colonial science chased after its own image of itself as able to know and control its subjects.

This chapter thus aims to speak to more than just the history of cartography. Colonialism is often seen as a project that sought to know its racial and environmental other through acts of classification, codification, and definition, which ultimately produced the certainties through which imperial rule could be effected. This chapter follows a broader shift within the medical humanities to deprivilege the study of knowing, and instead begin to look at the ways in which ignorance and uncertainty might be seen to have their own histories.[14] I, therefore, ask how we might begin to think about maps – quintessential tools of certainty – as records and of doubt and indecision. The maps that I discuss in this chapter fretfully mimicked the purported ability of colonial science to *know* its racial and social other, and the trace that they leave is thus one of uncertainty.

## The arrival of plague in India, 1896

The bubonic plague epidemic in India was part of a broader global event that is nowadays referred to as the third plague pandemic. The disease most probably emerged in Southern China in the late nineteenth century, and the first outbreak to come to widespread international attention was in Hong Kong in 1894. There for the first time in history, the bubonic plague was investigated through the new science of bacteriology. This work was carried out with an urgency resulting from the disease's mythic status as the medieval Black Death. As Christos Lynteris has observed, 'plague was thus rendered an object of knowledge under the bane of its perceived ability to wipe out humanity'.[15] During the Hong Kong outbreak, several bacteriologists competed to discover the microbial cause of the disease, with the Pasteurian Alexandre Yersin eventually identifying the plague bacterium, hence its modern scientific name, *Yersinia pestis*. Yersin's discovery did not, however, do much to demystify the disease, for the bacteriologist's new-found ability to know plague in the laboratory created further new uncertainties about how the disease spread from person to person. Major plague outbreaks on every inhabited continent in the decade following the first case in Hong Kong therefore often confused and bewildered sanitarians, who turned to a variety of techniques and technologies to both control and understand the disease. Both insanitary built environments and racialised others came under suspicion of spreading this feared disease. In Honolulu, for example, quarantine, inspection, and disinfection were supplemented by the burning of many Chinese-owned properties, which in January 1900 led to the accidental incineration of almost the entirety of the city's Chinatown.[16]

Bubonic plague arrived in Bombay in late 1896. The British reaction to the disease was bifurcated: on the one hand, the authorities expressed confidence that immediate and far-reaching sanitary measures could promptly bring the disease under control. At the same time, plague precipitated a panic among both the administration and the general population.[17] By January 1897, close to half the Indian population of Bombay had fled the city, causing major economic concerns for both the government and industrialists.[18] As one historian has recently argued, by 1897 the Bombay plague was, for legislators and officials, both a 'nightmare of death', and a fertile ground for the exercise of 'fantasies of social control'. Moreover, because neither the nature of the disease nor the appropriate control measures could be agreed upon in these early days of the epidemic, 'plague control had of necessity to be experimental'.[19] For all that was known about plague from the laboratory, its movement through the city confounded doctors, and it seemed to challenge cherished certainties that the British administration relied upon to control their Indian subjects. Plague spreads through human populations via a complicated pathway involving rodent hosts and insect vectors, none of which became known until the first decade of the twentieth century. In the final years of the nineteenth century, the unpredictable nature of the disease and the fact that it did not spread in an obvious fashion among what the British understood as insanitary subjects was thus a cause of much perplexity.[20] This was an uncertainty that continued to haunt plague science in India for at least the first decade of the epidemic.[21]

In this situation of uncertainty, the desire to control plague and the desire to know plague were wholly interlinked. This can be best understood from the enormous paper output produced by the government as a response to the plague. Between September 1896, when the first bubonic plague case was diagnosed in Bombay, and 1900, a series of reports, texts, and statements were published, which attempted to order plague through chronological accounts and to capture the nature of the epidemic through exhaustive detail.[22] In these lengthy and verbose narrative accounts, the unknown aetiology of the disease was discussed, while the efforts of the government to control it – which were only ever partially effective – were celebrated. In the appendices of these reports were maps that situated the disease in urban space. I investigate the way in which these reports related to these maps, and how the interaction between the two produced fantasies about how both the city and the plague might be known.

That these maps were produced in India was no coincidence. Around the world, the vast majority of plague outbreaks during the Third Pandemic were relatively contained events, and yet in India, the disease became endemic, recrudescing in the colder months of each year such that by 1930 it had killed more than 12 million people in the country.[23] The initial confidence felt by the British administration that they could control the plague soon disappeared, and what replaced it was an urgent desire to understand the confusing spread of this disease.

## The creation of the Plague Committee

In the late nineteenth century, the Indian government was as a rule committed to a non-interventionist, hands-off approach to infectious disease outbreaks such as smallpox and cholera.[24] Plague, however, occupied a special case, as its feared and much-mythologised history drove an unprecedented level of state intervention. As the historian David Arnold has shown, this intervention frequently preceded the arrival of the disease, and for the Indian population, was often 'far more distressing' than the actual epidemic.[25] Sanitary activity began in October 1896, with enforced segregation, hospitalisation, and urban cleansing.[26] It nonetheless quickly became clear that such measures were having little effect on the spread of plague, and consequently, the government hastily introduced new legislation – the Epidemic Diseases Act of February 1897 – which gave the authorities almost unlimited power to do whatever needed to halt the disease across the whole of India. In Bombay, the passing of this Act led to the creation of a Plague Committee with powers to supersede the Municipal Corporation of the city in all matters relating to plague. With no clear idea of how to rid the city of disease, this Committee continued and intensified the already existing sanitary programme of highly intrusive plague measures involving house-to-house inspections, compulsory disinfection, and forced patient removal. These measures were not guided by any uniform theory of the disease. Borrowing Michael Worboys' terms, these sanitary policies consisted of 'exclusive' interventions such as isolation and targeted disinfection, but implemented in a scattered and chaotic fashion that harked back to 'inclusive' sanitary policies that saw the city as space of danger and infection.[27] These sanitary policies were, in other words, directed by no single epistemological understanding of plague, but aimed to halt the disease in any way possible.

The exhaustive nature of the Plague Committee's sanitary measures were exceeded only by the comprehensive manner in which they were documented and recorded. In 1897, under the direction of its chairman, Brigadier-General W. F. Gatacre, the Committee narrated its activities during the first plague season in a painstakingly thorough report, the main volume of which stretched over 258 pages.[28] Much of this report was devoted to the minutiae of the sanitary process:

the organisation and management of personnel; the arrangement of camps and hospitals; the routines of duty. It was also in large part a justification for measures that had frequently aroused intense opposition and resentment from local populations. The job of the Committee had never been to determine the bacteriological and clinical nature of plague – that task had been assigned to other functionaries, mainly within the Indian Medical Service.[29] Nonetheless, the Committee's report speculated extensively on the nature of plague. Among wide-ranging observations of plague's clinical signs (for example, descriptions of the 'earthy, clear-like odour' coming from patients' skin and breath),[30] extensive patient case studies, and descriptions of individual symptoms, the report also asked questions about, for example, why the disease was infectious in the city but not in hospitals.[31] The best answer that could be given was that plague became contagious in insanitary conditions, and thus within a sanitary hospital, remained non-infectious.

What is most remarkable about this report is that just as the Committee described how they had attempted to control the plague through recourse to multiple rationalities, theories and methods – in other words, *in any way possible* – so too did they appear to be willing to try and understand the disease *in any way possible*. Take, for example, a section of the report, by a Dr A. McCabe Dallas, which recounted the 'statistical and clinical record of work done' in Bombay's Grant Road Hospital. Before reaching the statistical and clinical evidence, Dallas gave an extensive account of his own understanding of plague's transmission. He argued that rats harboured the infection and caused it to multiply. He argued that drains too were implicated, due to being contaminated by matter coming from infected patients. Soil was also seen as a dangerous location of infection, particularly sewage soil, and Dallas was extremely complimentary about sanitary measures to flush sewers with disinfectant. He also, however, argued that the disease was airborne: micro-organisms escaping from decomposing rats would ascend with hot air currents and thus travel across a locality. Other forms of transmission that Dallas considered included the sharing of drinking vessels. Pneumonic plague, he concluded, was the only form of the disease directly transmitted by human intercourse.[32]

Many of Dallas' speculations aligned with areas of investigation that would give way to a much more comprehensive understanding of plague in the coming decades. What is striking about his reasoning, however, is that it embraced a multiplicity of factors and a multiplicity of possible ways in which plague could be understood to spread across the city. No single cause was given weight – instead, every possible avenue of transmission was considered as a potential mode through which plague could propagate. The Plague Committee's 'inclusive' inclinations in sanitation were thus echoed in their multifactorial accounts of the disease; to borrow a phrase from Worboys, this was a report that was more concerned 'not to be wrong than to risk being right'.[33] This report, in other words, sought every possible avenue through which truth about plague might be spoken: in a situation of radical uncertainty about the sanitary future of the city, it cast as wide a net as possible in order to try and catch some truth about the disease.

It is in light of this encompassing search for certain knowledge that attempts to map the Bombay plague have to be understood. The Bombay plague outbreak occurred at a particular moment in colonial medicine, when medical geography, once the 'queen of the medical sciences' was slowly giving way to a new scientific medicine of laboratories and bacteriology.[34] Not only did the new science of bacteriology lead to a de-privileging of the map, but it also led to a slow transformation in which theories of disease moved away from environmental and spatial forms of reasoning. As Warwick Anderson has shown, bacteriology wrought a transformation in the tropics such that imaginaries of problematic environs eventually gave way to the idea of dangerous germ-carrying native bodies. This was, however, an extremely slow process, and as bacteriology first rose to prominence it served rather to 'adjust or extend' preceding theories of geographic pathology.[35] In other words – as has been shown so many times in relation to this epidemic – the bacteriological 'revolution' in plague was slow and uneven.[36]

This slow and uneven adjustment was particularly noticeable in the early years of the Bombay plague. A partial bacteriological understanding of the plague epidemic frequently obscured the disease for colonial observers, for its indirect mode of transmission did not seem to fit with accepted understandings of bacterial disease. As a result, theories of environmental propagation were frequently added to notions of bacterial transmission, to create what historians have described as a theory of 'contingent contagion', that is, an understanding that plague was passed between bodies but also encouraged by environments.[37] Such notions fell comfortably within an Anglo-Indian medical tradition, which during the late nineteenth century was often famously resistant to contagionist thinking.[38] For many of India's late nineteenth-century doctors, germ theory could provide only a partial explanation for diseases that they viewed as primarily environmental.[39]

In such a situation, where laboratory discoveries only seemed to further mystify the disease, and where germ theory was not trusted to give a full account of an epidemic, medical cartography continued to be seen as a form of reasoning that could persuasively fashion arguments beyond the laboratory. In this regard, the maps contained within the Committee's report represented an important hope: they were spaces of exploration in which a *certain* plague science could be imagined and made possible.

The rest of this chapter asks how our analysis might be enhanced if we begin to think of maps of the Bombay plague not just as records of the disease, but as objects of attraction and desire. In doing this, I follow recent developments in the history of science that have embraced anthropological approaches to documents as material objects – 'paper technologies' – that can perform social and political functions.[40] These plague maps were, I argue, spaces of desire that stood in a particular physical relationship to an archive of reports that otherwise aspired to narrate the plague in its totality. As complicated images that were printed on large sheets of paper, the maps were often physically separate from or additional to the volumes they accompanied. There was a straightforward technical reason for this, for these maps were irregular and hard to print. This chapter, however, seeks to interrogate the question of the distance between text and map in order to ask how the supplementary nature of these maps as 'paperwork' contributed to their authority.[41] How is it that having a relationship to text that was never quite stable led to these maps having an imitative truthfulness? Within the archive of plague, the map was an interesting technology, for it was of necessity supplementary and separate from text, and yet it was also the place where colonial science promised and suggested forms of argument that could achieve a synthesis of data instead of an excess of information.

My goal is thus to contribute to the history of the medical geography of plague by showing how an investigation of the tensions between text and map can uncover fantasies and longings within colonial medicine's engagement with the city. As arguments, these maps might be thought of as deceptions. They posed as arguments and they carried the visual rhetoric of an argument, but they were simulacra of arguments; mimetic hints at the possibility of arguments. This chapter considers a moment in medical geography when the power of the map to argue was already an object of desire. The maps analysed here were thus statements, not so much of how things were, but of how things were desired to be. My analysis takes in three case studies. The first two maps were created early in the epidemic, and represent attempts to grasp plague at both micro and macro levels. The final case study is from 1914, at a point when plague had been stabilised as an epistemic object.

## Three case studies

### 1. Worli Koliwada

The city of Bombay presented a challenge to plague research, due to its population of nearly 850,000, its mobile residents, its rapid development, and its heterogeneous composition.[42] The Plague Committee, therefore, focused upon specific micro-examples in order to gain a better understanding of the efficacy of sanitary policy within Bombay. I here examine a case study contained in the Committee's report, one of a number of such studies of urban villages spread throughout the peninsula, each of which was accompanied by a map.

One of these villages, Worli Koliwada (fishing village), had a peripheral relationship to the city that surrounded it, being a self-contained settlement on the northern peninsula of one of the original seven islands of Bombay. The Committee chose to study plague in Worli partly because the disease was uncharacteristically virulent there, with over 90 per cent of those infected dying in a few hours.[43] Plague is manifested in three main forms: bubonic, pneumonic, and much more rarely, septicemic. If the Committee's statistics were accurate, they point towards pneumonic infection, which is an airborne disease, spread directly and rapidly from person to person. No mention, however, was made in the report as to the predominant type of plague present in Worli.

Worli village was also chosen for study because of its relative isolation from the rest of the district, and its seemingly stable population. For the Committee, it must have appeared as a manageable and controllable case. There was, additionally, a degree of autonomous organisation in the village that attracted the Committee. The report noted with approval that the villagers had from the outset been 'fully alive to the dangers' of the disease, and consequently, they had decided at the very beginning of the epidemic to place watchmen at the entrances to their village. These guards both prevented strangers from entering and prevented villagers from leaving to visit stricken parts of the city. This spontaneous sanitary cordon was nonetheless ultimately unsuccessful, and the first case of plague appeared in the village on 1 December 1896.[44]

At a basic level, the Committee's report on Worli was a narrative of disinfection operations within the village, embedded within a larger chapter detailing sanitary activities in Bombay, such as house-to-house visitation and disinfection. The report's authors did not, however, limit themselves to simple narration. They also speculated upon the spread of plague. In doing so, they adopted a style of writing in which knowing plague, controlling it, and describing it were intimately related practices. In this way, the report was saturated by multiple possible explanations for the plague, each of which was nonetheless inconclusive. The report made reference to the dark and low huts of the residents, the lack of artificial drainage, and the narrow streets that nonetheless benefitted from sea-breezes on both sides.[45] It described how the ground of the village was receptive to plague due to the 'drainage of generations' soaking into the soil, and the villagers letting their water flow into that ground.[46] It described in detail the disinfecting operations, in which 270 coolies were employed in an operation that involved removing the roof from every single house in the village, in the belief that enabling sunlight and fresh air to enter the houses would purify them of plague. The supposed success of this measure again implied the possibility of an understanding of the disease as something that could adhere to the material structure of the city and then subsequently infect humans. Worli, as with many other localities in Bombay, was seen as so dangerous that a wholesale disinfection of the entire village was understood to be necessary.

Within the Committee's description of this fishing village, multiple possibilities of knowing plague were considered: none were wholly conclusive. Nonetheless, the report did promise its readers a certain understanding about plague, not in its own pages, but within a map that lay in a physically separate volume.

This map is shown in Figure 5.1. For the authors of the report, the map threw light 'on the way in which the disease spreads'.[47] The map was a detailed tracing of the outline of all 936 mud houses in Worli, which at the beginning of the epidemic were home to 5,493 people. These houses were individually numbered and then plague cases were drawn by hand in three groupings. The first grouping, in red, consisted of a single case. The second grouping (in yellow) contained four further cases, and the third grouping (in green) consisted of all other plague cases. These corresponded to the chart beneath showing plague cases against time. Additionally, this chart indicated the dates upon which sanitary operations were begun and completed. For the authors of the report, the grouping of these cases appeared to promise an understanding of plague. Precisely what this understanding could be, however, was deferred to the map, in other words, to a space beyond the text.

The map was nonetheless riven by a tension, for it was being called upon to function as both a demonstration of disinfection operations in Worli and as evidence of the epidemic's spread. It was, in other words, being made to simultaneously make an argument about aetiology and about the efficiency of colonial policy. Ultimately, in its peculiar visual composition, it provided a vision of the city as a place of almost endless disease potentiality that was uninterrogated, unspecific and in many ways unknown. As already explained, the report itself envisioned the ground of the city – clogged by human effluvia and wastewater – as a fertile space of plague possibilities. In the map of Worli, only houses and built structures were made to stand out in relief, making the map an unusual representation of urban space in that it showed units of habitation, but not roads or streets through which movement or flow could occur. The result was that the ground of the village was coterminous with the paper of the map, and was bisected only by a single line to indicate the Eastern shore of the peninsula. At the top of the map (to the west) the ground spread out, city became paper and vice versa: this was a fecund surface of undifferentiated disease possibility. Within this map, the ground of the city was thus equated with plague, in such a way as to create a bewilderment of possibilities. The map could not, however, reveal the details of transmission that the Committee so sorely sought to know.

The centrality of idioms of flow and movement to the construction of an ideal sanitary city in the early twentieth century is well documented in contemporary urban studies,[48] and in post-plague Bombay, visions of unrestricted flow came to dominate plans for urban renewal, even if they were not always realised.[49] Here, however, flow was understood as a property of the insanitary city: this map pictured disease flowing across the surface of the urban in an unimpeded fashion.

The Worli map was not alone. A similar relationship between text and map can be seen in multiple other case studies from the Committee's report. The report contained three further maps of other urban villages in Bombay: Sewri Koliwada, Parel Village, and Mahim Koliwada. As with the map of Worli, these showed plague cases arranged by colour in groups and placed in numbered houses, corresponding to tables charting deaths by time. Taken together, these plans showed little evidence for the success of disinfection, for where disinfection correlated with a diminishing of plague (as in Worli and Sewri) there were also widespread exoduses from the villages, as terrified residents fled the epidemic. In each case, the text gave way to speculation about infection by suggesting that these maps be taken as evidence of the grouping of cases and as evidence of personal infection, while also continuing to point towards the expansive ground of these villages as sources of filth and disease. In each case, an attempt to understand was deferred to the promise that the map would provide understanding.

In these narrative accounts of plague in the urban villages of Bombay, the map was thus continually invoked as a synthesiser. The maps were presented as promises to speak with certainty about the grouping of cases and the relationships

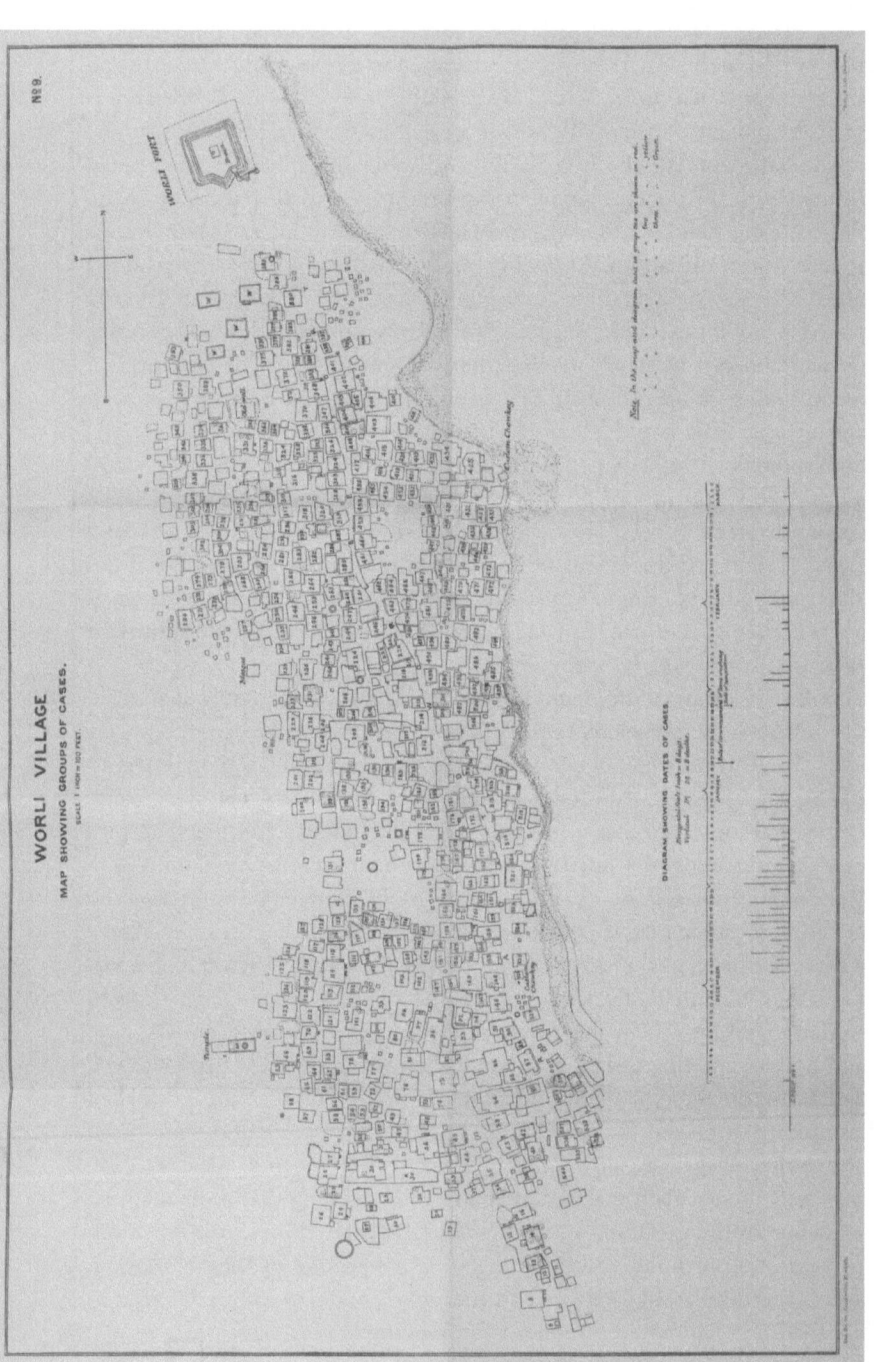

**FIGURE 5.1** Map of Worli Village, originally from the *Report on the Bubonic Plague in Bombay* by the Plague Committee. This image is of a reproduction of the original, in: R. Nathan *The Plague in India*, 1898. The reproduction differs from the original on two points only: the orientation has been changed (north–south is now horizontal) and the bar chart has been placed below the map rather than on a different page . Reproduced by kind permission of the Syndics of Cambridge University Library; V.10.90

between them. In each of these short village studies, the report assured its readers that they would find an argument in the corresponding map, but this posed a problem. The report as a whole was simply too multifactorial to ever give a clear account of the disease: that is, it tended to see every factor as a potential cause of plague in such a way that no single factor could ever be a certain cause. Its assumptions about what plague could be and from whence plague could emerge were so all-embracing that no clear relationship between place and body as mediated by disease could ever be suggested. This report could not say how plague related within and through the urban because it ultimately ended up equating the disease *with* the urban. Each of the village case studies nonetheless promised to answer specific questions about the relationships between plague cases by reference to maps. These maps can, therefore, be seen as fantasy-spaces in which desires for comprehension could be deposited. Here we can see what Harley described as the 'charisma' of the map: the idea that through its technical precision, the map might precisely mirror the world as it really is.[50]

In summarising nineteenth-century debates surrounding cholera, Tom Koch tells us how 'the wealth of data was too complex for a simple inductive argument, too vast for a simple statement'.[51] Mapping thus became an 'essential medium' through which such data could be 'transformed into arguments'.[52] The Plague Committee's maps must be understood against such a moment in medical history when maps were seen as capable of transforming data into reason. The maps in this report, however, did not do this. Instead, they mimicked this capability.

## 2. Situating plague on the map

As has been seen, the surface of the city appeared as a particularly problematic object for colonial science. The fact that this surface was seen as a fecund layer out of which plague could emerge was behind much of the colonial uncertainty about the disease. The surface of the city, in other words, appeared to be so ripe with the potential for disease that any simple explanation of this disease was precluded. The ground, the soil, surface water, the floors of houses, the coating of walls, and the roofs of dwellings were all implicated in the transmission of plague and were all objects of sanitary intervention – being either destroyed or disinfected by the Plague Committee's gangs of coolies and soldiers.[53] The Committee desired to both know and control the surface of the city. In this context, the map of Worli carried a promise of a clear understanding of plague, but it too ultimately produced an image of the city's surface as unknowable, uncontrollable, and subject to an unlimited flow of plague. The Worli map thus emerged as a space of desire; desire both for a way to argue plague and desire for a legible surface to the city.

A year after the publication of the Plague Committee's report, in 1898, the Worli map and case study were reprinted in another multi-volume report about the plague in the Bombay Presidency.[54] Compiled by the civil servant Robert Nathan, this report was an attempt to narrate plague as a totality that comprised both the story of the epidemic and the story of the government's response. Statements from various texts and other sources were collected and placed together to give a narrative of the disease that was both historical and geographic. It was an accumulation of all possible ways of describing plague, and thus, like the Committee's report, it was characterised by a structural glut of data that rendered impossible any conclusion. Included in this report were a number of maps, one of which can be seen in Figure 5.2. This map depicted the 'principal places where plague was endemic' in the Bombay Presidency. It did so through the combination of two elements: a standard survey-map of the territory overlain by a series of dots that had been added to indicate cities where plague was epidemic.

The map in Figure 5.2 elucidated two important features of Nathan's report. Firstly, as with the Worli map, this map was physically separate from the text of the report and promised a certainty that could not be found within his prose. This map was one of a series that, for Nathan, stood in the place of a description of the 'course' that plague took in the Bombay Presidency. Textual description was unnecessary, he explained, for the statements, maps, and charts in the appendices 'furnish as clear a picture of the epidemic as any verbal description could convey'.[55] The statements that he referred to consisted of twenty-five pages of statistics: reports on plague seizures (sudden attacks of illness) and deaths; comparisons of weakly mortalities; a statement that set seizures against temperature and humidity.[56] In this context, the disease maps were once again being asked to function so as to translate an excess of data into something readable.[57] The clarity that Nathan lauded was quite clearly not to be found in the charts and statements, but rather in the maps that synthesised them. Figure 5.2 was thus presented as an orphan argument parallel to Nathan's account that stood in lieu of text and made legible a set of otherwise impenetrable charts. Yet in spite of Nathan's seeming confidence in the explanatory possibility of his charts, the map itself was ineffectual as an argument, for it made no conjectures about relations in a way that could explain disease. Nathan's map spoke neither of temporal relations nor of relations of intensity or contact. This is not, however, to say that relations were absent from the map, for it established in forceful terms a relationship between the plotting of plague and another potent form of colonial control: the cartographic depiction of space.

This brings us to the second important feature of Figure 5.2: it can be seen as an attempt to respond to that central problem of plague: the seeming illegibility of the surface of the city. This becomes clear when we look at how this map was constructed. It was based upon a plan of the Bombay Presidency from the office of the Surveyor-General, complete with lines of latitude and longitude, and details of railways up until 1894. This was a map produced out of a colonial survey of the country: a map that was designed to demonstrate a grasp of imperial territory, and which promised 'the potential perfection of the map's relationship with the territory mapped'.[58] It was a perfect example of the 'mimetic map', which could claim to '*be* the territory' it represented.[59] As such, it was part of a cartographic archive, which for the British was a 'perfect geographic panopticon'.[60] In Figure 5.2, plague had therefore been superimposed upon an archetypal image of colonial control. In this map, the surface and ground of the territory had been transformed into an

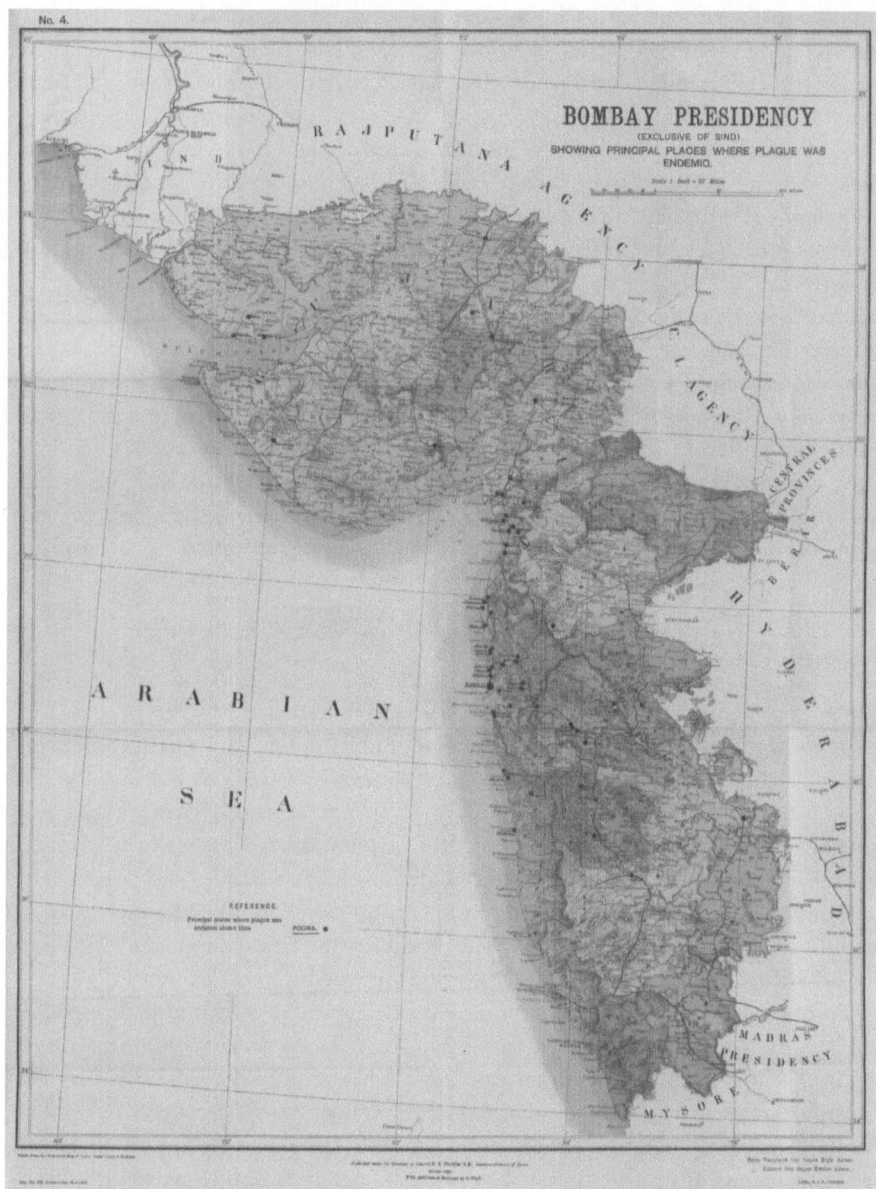

**FIGURE 5.2**  Bombay Presidency (exclusive of Sind): map showing the principal places where plague was endemic, in: R. Nathan, *The Plague in India, 1898.* Reproduced by kind permission of the Syndics of Cambridge University Library; V.10.90

eminently knowable and legible representation, and plague had been placed atop of this. This map, therefore, offered up a possibility of both knowing and controlling disease in the same way that the British understood themselves to know and control the landscape of India. Contained in this map was a longing for the plague administrator's knowledge to be as sure and complete as the (already mythical) knowledge of the surveyor. What is once again obvious is the desire to incorporate the mythic explanatory power of the map into an uncertain plague science: Figure 5.2's power lay in its ability to ape and conjure a regime of visual authority.

As the anthropologist Matthew Hull has argued, there has long been a poverty to our understanding of maps 'as the most basic technology and most fundamental metaphor of modern state surveillance and control'.[61] For Hull, anti-positivist approaches to maps have often underplayed the map's referential function and thus obscured the fact that the map's ideological work is bound up 'in the practices that link maps to the realities they reference'.[62] How might we build upon such work to understand the way in which the ideological power of a map can be bound up in its referencing of a larger genre of mapping? This map of plague in the Bombay Presidency gained its power not so much through its claims to represent a spatial reality, but rather through its mimetic evocation of a genre that was seen to control space with exactitude. Understanding this helps us to appreciate that the weakness of some maps is not only, as Matthew Edney has argued, their disorder and partiality, but also the fact that they represent the repugnant other of colonialism: the 'bad copy'.[63]

## 3. Erasing the city's surface

The map in Figure 5.2 was not an isolated example: rather it was part of a broader fantasy within colonial science that plague might be known if only the problematic surface of the city could be erased. A good example of this can be found in the musings of the Bombay Health Officer, J. A. Turner, in 1903. Turner's quarterly sanitary reports make interesting reading, for he often treated them almost as a personal diary: a space to criticise the short-sightedness of colleagues and to speculate on ways to improve the sanitary condition of the city. One wonders whether he thought anybody was reading them. His report for the first quarter of 1903 is particularly utopian in its speculations about the sanitary future of Bombay.[64]

Turner began this quarterly report with a reiteration of the idea that plague had become a disease of locality. Plague had recrudesced every winter since 1896, and it was now clearly endemic in Bombay. What is more, he lamented that few scientific advances had been made in understanding this disease since 1897. The disease, Turner argued, was clearly communicable between persons, and between persons and rats. But, he claimed, it was almost certainly also to be found within the fabric of the city. Like so many of his contemporaries, Turner thus transposed a germ theory of plague onto an older view that saw the disease as imbricated in the material space of the city.[65] For Turner, this conclusion meant that sanitary improvement would be impossible without years of disruption and rebuilding. Turner's response to this – his utopian dream – was of a city without a surface; a space of figure but no ground; a space in which dirt could not linger.

Beginning his reverie with the words 'but supposing it were possible . . .', Turner proposed the creation of a floating city of 300,000 people in the Back Bay of Bombay. Constructed out of floating houses and piers, this temporary structure would, he conjectured, provide lodging for the city's day labourers while giving them quick and easy access to their places of employment in the south of the city. It would expose them to ample fresh air and sunlight, and water for washing would be plentiful. More importantly, it would create a space for total surveillance; workers moving back and forth between the floating city and their work on land would be under constant observation, 'every case of sickness reported and every death verified'. To remove the people from the surface of the city was therefore also to make them and their diseases observable and controllable in a way that had never been possible before. Furthermore, Turner argued that the creation of this floating utopia would enable improvements on shore: filthy houses could be demolished, streets cleaned, and most importantly, soil in the infected parts of the city would be able to dry out. All of this could be achieved because a city with a porous and therefore dangerous ground would be replaced by a city with no ground at all.

Turner's idea ultimately had no afterlife; it was a thought experiment buried within his normal work reports. It nonetheless tells us what it meant to dream of controllable, *knowable*, plague in 1903. It meant imagining a city in which there was, quite literally, no ground and no surface. We have already seen from the Worli village map that the problem of *knowing* plague was tied to its excessive spread across the ground of the city. In Figure 5.2, this problematic ground was replaced by a surface of trigonometric certainty. Turner's musings represented a third response to this same dilemma, but one in which the problematic ground or surface of the city was discarded in favour of the purifying instability of water. Much has been written of imperial desires for a colony without people, particularly in relation to colonial visual culture's habit of emptying lands of natives.[66] Here, by contrast, we see a desire for a colony of productive native labour, shorn of the territory in which they lived.

Turner's utopian musings came at the end of the period of plague science characterised by radical uncertainty. Specifically, new and very specific understandings of the disease began to percolate in the Indian medical establishment after 1906, when a new Plague Commission was instituted in India as a joint venture between the Government of India, the Royal Society, and the Lister Institute.[67] This Commission carried out both large-scale epidemiological work and laboratory studies, which primarily focused upon understanding the role of plague's hosts and vectors. This led to significant advances being made in the understanding of plague as a zoonotic disease, and plague ceased to be seen as a troubling disease of locality. Concern shifted from the environment to infected bodies, both human and animal, and plague mapping consequently decreased in frequency and importance. The use of maps as spaces of epidemiological theorisation and argumentation continued sporadically until the end of the decade, but they were slowly supplanted by other methods.[68] This was part of a more general trend: the maps discussed in this chapter stood at the very end of a long period when medical geography was felt to contribute significantly to the progress of medical science.[69] By the late 1910s, plague publications from India increasingly used maps only to orientate readers to place. These maps showed where things had happened but had no overlay of disease: there was no longer any attempt to create a relationship between the disease and the space thus depicted.[70] More broadly, multi-causal explanations and expansive narratives that sought to assess the character of the disease were abandoned in favour of accounts that focused upon the mechanisms of plague's spread between human and animal bodies.[71]

Yet it was in this later stage of plague science that we can observe the emergence of a form of mapping – and I use the term in its loosest sense – that most clearly realised Turner's fantasy. The most striking example of this can be found in Figure 5.3, which has been taken from a paper about the bionomics of the common rat flea, published by the Indian Plague Commission in 1914.[72] At this point, the role of the flea as a vector of bubonic plague was well established. The Indian Plague Commission were thus conducting experiments to try and understand everything they possibly could about the flea's life history so as to better ascertain the insect's role in communicating the disease. Figure 5.3 is the end product of an experiment to try and establish the ability of newly hatched flea larvae to survive without food. To do this, a number of rat and human flea larvae were placed in test tubes and left without food to see how they would survive in different temperature and humidity conditions. The 'crawling powers' of freshly emerged unfed larvae were then put to the test. The larvae were placed at the centre of white sheets of paper on which various other substances – blood-stained

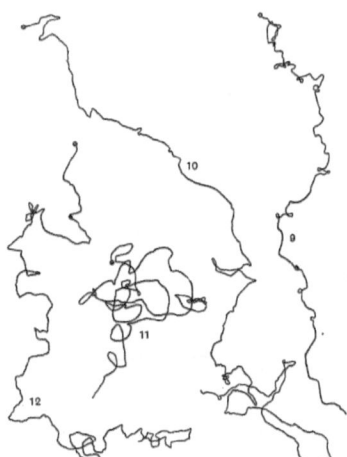
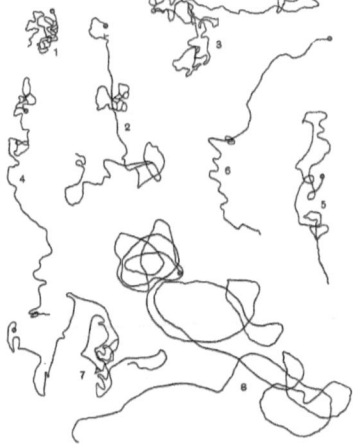

FIGURE 5.3   Bombay Presidency (exclusive of Sind): the map-in-miniature showing the effacement of the surface, in: A. Bacot, 'LXIX. A study of the bionomics of the common rat fleas and other species associated with human habitations, with special reference to the influence of temperature and humidity at various periods of the life history of the insect', *The Journal of Hygiene*, 13 (1914), 447–654

rags, flea faeces, plain cloth, and sand – had been arranged at equal distances from their starting point. The movement of each larva was then followed with a pencil for thirty minutes. This test failed to produce the results the experimenters had hoped for – that the larvae would show an inclination to seek out food. The tracings were nonetheless used to create the two maps-in-miniature that make up Figure 5.3. The lines, produced by the tracing of the pencil, were rearranged in relation to one another in order to fit upon the paper. When we think about the technicalities of this operation, we realise that the multiple invisible backgrounds (that is, the very pieces of paper) upon which the larvae crawled had to be quite literally cut up and stitched together in order to produce these miniature pathways. Multiple events were placed upon a single plane in a process that completely obliterated the surfaces upon which the crawling occurred. An exact, specific detail of the bionomics of a single plague vector thus came to be known, but in doing so the ground upon which it occurred was erased.

In some ways, this map-in-miniature achieved what the other maps could not; a complete erasure of a surface, whose relationship to plague produced excesses that undermined colonial attempts to know and to control. This map's condition of existence was the literal destruction of the *ground* upon which it was built. It was, in miniature form, the achievement of Turner's fantasy.

In many ways, this echoes histories of clinical photography in this period. For example, Ari Larissa Heinrich has shown how racial tensions played out in clinical photography at the turn of the twentieth century in China, where contextual and biographical data about Chinese subjects was over time edited out of clinical photographs, until finally the Chinese subject entirely vanished 'from the image to which it has become essentially superfluous'.[73] The racialised body and, in this case, the tumour, were separated from one another, prompting Heinrich to ask a question that might be applied to these Indian plague maps: when plague was totally separated from the surface of the city, 'we know only that there was a pathology and that the pathology has been removed. The question is, which one?'[74] For British doctors, it was the Indian city, and not the disease, which posed the real diagnostic questions. The maps examined in this chapter promised an understanding of that city, but only when the city was expunged could they make comprehensible arguments about disease.

## Rethinking the mimetic map

In this chapter, I have examined the medical cartography of the Bombay plague in order to explore an ambiguous relationship between actual certainty and the desire for certainty. In doing this, I have argued for an expanded reading of the mimetic map: these are maps that functioned by imitating the certainty that their makers attributed to cartography as a genre.

More broadly, it is perhaps time that we began to think seriously about the ways in which the desire for certainty is embedded within our understanding of disease maps. A good example of why this is necessary can be taken from Kari

McLeod's analysis of the most famous of all disease maps: John Snow's 1854 dot-map of cholera.[75] Snow drew this map during a debilitating outbreak of cholera in London's Soho. The dot-map is much celebrated by modern medical geography, as it is seen as a crucial tool through which Snow was able to arrive at the conclusion that cholera was spreading from the contaminated water of a single pump. Based on this information, Snow removed the handle from the pump and thus ended the outbreak. Perhaps no medical map is more famous, and it is a factor in Snow's modern reputation as a hero of epidemiology. Recent reappraisals, however, have questioned the importance of the map to Snow's epidemiological reasoning. McLeod has shown that Snow's dot-map has been subject to much memorialisation within medical geography, even though there is little archival evidence to support the idea that Snow actually used the map to determine the source of the cholera outbreak. Indeed, Snow's textual references to the map are almost entirely descriptive. In spite of this, the dot-map has become a mythologised example of the power of medical cartography to reveal what cannot be seen by other methods. Examining the legacy of this map, McLeod asks whether disease maps always show causation or prove anything. 'Do medical cartographers actually state that causation and proof exist in their maps, or do the map interpreters project those expectations?'[76]

To respond to such a question requires that we understand the forms of legitimisation and authority that exist between and within genres of reasoning in a paper archive. This chapter has attempted to do just that: I have argued that to fully understand practices of disease mapping in late nineteenth-century India, we have to understand the attraction of mapping as a genre that seemed to promise certainty. When the authors of reports on plague referred to maps, they were not just engaging in forms of reasoning, but also attempting to capture a way of knowing that seemed elusive and impossible. I have, in other words, attempted to show how recourses to mapping in plague science were often attempts to mimic other, more certain forms of knowledge and control. In particular, I have shown how, in the Bombay plague, disease maps were an imitative attempt to capture the promised certainty of their own genre.

What are the advantages of thinking about mapping as a genre that could sometimes imitate its own power to make arguments? For a start, this approach can begin to challenge narratives of plague in India as a series of competing claims made by physicians and administrators with absolute certainty. Furthermore, it can help us to uncover the tensions and desires that suffused a situation of radical uncertainty and ignorance. It helps us to understand why histories of certainty are often more tempting to write than histories of unknowing, for these maps always presented themselves *as if they were* arguments springing from certitude. If we want to understand the ways in which plague and the city were thought to relate to one another in maps, then we must understand the relationship between maps as paper objects and the wider archive to which they belonged. As objects, these maps could be spaces of desirous thinking about plague in Bombay, but as instruments of colonial science, they only imitated forms of power and control.

# Notes

1 Research leading to this chapter was funded by the European Research Council Starting Grant under the European Union's Seventh Framework Programme/ERC grant agreement no. 336564; European Research Council [FP7/2007–2013] for the project Visual Representations of the Third Plague Pandemic (CRASSH, University of Cambridge).
2 Koch, 'Knowing Its Place'.
3 *Ibid., Disease Maps*, 12.
4 *Ibid.*, 116.
5 Harley, 'Deconstructing the Map'.
6 Edney, *Mapping an Empire*, 332.
7 Harley, 'Historical Geography and the Cartographic Illusion', 83.
8 Evans, 'Blaming the Rat? Accounting for Plague in Colonial Indian Medicine'.
9 Harley, 'Historical Geography and the Cartographic Illusion', 83.
10 *Ibid.*, 83.
11 Taussig, *Mimesis and Alterity*.
12 Published in multiple volumes between 1890 and 1915, this is often taken to be the foundational text in British Social Anthropology.
13 Taussig, *Shamanism*.
14 For example, Proctor and Schiebinger, *Agnotology*; Samimian-Darash and Rabinow, *Modes of Uncertainty*.
15 Lynteris, *Ethnographic Plague*, 1.
16 Echenberg, *Plague Ports*, 198–202; Mohr, *Plague and Fire*.
17 Chandavarkar, 'Plague Panic and Epidemic Politics in India, 1896–1914'.
18 Sarkar, 'The Tie That Snapped'.
19 *Ibid.*, 184.
20 Evans, 'Blaming the Rat? Accounting for Plague in Colonial Indian Medicine'.
21 Hankin, 'On the Epidemiology of Plague'.
22 Campbell and Mostyn, *Report of the Bombay Plague Committee*; Gatacre, *Report on the Bubonic Plague*; Nathan, *The Plague in India, 1896, 1897*.
23 Arnold, *Colonizing the Body*, 202.
24 *Ibid.*, 203.
25 *Ibid.*, 202.
26 *Ibid.*, 203–204.
27 Worboys, *Spreading Germs*.
28 Gatacre, *Report on the Bubonic Plague*.
29 Report by Surgeon Major R. W. S. Lyons, I. M. S., President of the Plague Research Committee. National Archives of India. Home: Sanitary Plague: B: August 1898: Nos. 96–98.
30 Gatacre, *Report on the Bubonic Plague*, 58.
31 *Ibid.*, 50–51.
32 *Ibid.*, 93–94.
33 Worboys, *Spreading Germs*, 120.
34 Numbers, 'Medical Science', 1.
35 Anderson, *Colonial Pathologies*, 24.
36 Peckham, 'Matshed Laboratory'; Sutphen, 'Not What, but Where'.
37 Prashant Kidambi, '"An Infection of Locality"'.
38 Harrison, 'A Question of Locality'.
39 Arnold, *Colonizing the Body*, 36.
40 Delbourgo and Müller-Wille, 'Introduction'; Müller-Wille and Charmantier, 'Lists as Research Technologies'.
41 Delbourgo and Müller-Wille, 'Introduction', 712.
42 On the population of the city, see Arnold, *Colonizing the Body*, 207.
43 Gatacre, *Report on the Bubonic Plague*, 187.
44 *Ibid.*, 188.

45  *Ibid.*, 187.
46  *Ibid.*, 188.
47  *Ibid.*
48  Sennett, *Flesh and Stone.*
49  Kidambi, *The Making of an Indian Metropolis.*
50  Harley, 'Historical Geography and the Cartographic Illusion', 82.
51  Koch, *Disease Maps*, 117.
52  *Ibid.*
53  For an examination of soil as 'an unstable yet highly productive epistemic thing' during the third plague pandemic, see Lynteris, '"Suitable Soil"', 343.
54  Nathan, *The Plague in India, 1896, 1897.*
55  *Ibid., Vol. I*, 95.
56  Nathan, *The Plague in India, 1896, 1897, Vol. II*, 109–134.
57  Koch, *Disease Maps*, 117.
58  Edney, *Mapping an Empire*, 21.
59  *Ibid.*, 21.
60  *Ibid.*, 34.
61  Hull, *Government of Paper*, 212.
62  *Ibid.*, 230.
63  Gable, 'Bad Copies'.
64  British Library, IOR/V/25/840/23, Health Officer's Report for the 1st Quarter of 1903.
65  Sutphen, 'Not What, but Where'.
66  See, for example, Ryan, *Picturing Empire.*
67  This is not to be confused with the 1900 Commission of Inquiry – the Fraser Commission – into plague in India.
68  For example, Anon., 'XXXV. On the Spread of Epidemic Plague'; Tucker, *The Management of a Plague Epidemic.*
69  Anderson, 'Geography, Race and Nation'; Numbers, 'Medical Science before Scientific Medicine'.
70  E.g. Kunhardt and Taylor, 'LXXII. Epidemiological Observations'; Gloster and White, 'LXXXIII. Epidemiological Observations'.
71  Evans, 'Blaming the Rat?'
72  Bacot, 'LXIX. A Study of the Bionomics'.
73  Heinrich, *The Afterlife of Images*, 111.
74  *Ibid.*
75  McLeod, 'Our Sense of Snow'.
76  *Ibid.*, 926.

## References

Anderson, Warwick, *Colonial Pathologies: American Tropical Medicine, Race, and Hygiene in the Philippines* (Durham: Duke University Press, 2006).

Anderson, Warwick, 'Geography, Race and Nation: Remapping "Tropical" Australia', 1890–1930, *Medical History*, 44, S20 (2000), 146–159.

Anon., 'XXXV. On the Spread of Epidemic Plague through Districts with Scattered Villages: With a Statistical Analysis by Dr M. Greenwood', *The Journal of Hygiene*, 10, 3 (1910), 349–445.

Arnold, David, *Colonizing the Body: State Medicine and Epidemic Disease in Nineteenth-Century India* (Berkeley: University of California Press, 1993).

Bacot, A., 'LXIX. A Study of the Bionomics of the Common Rat Fleas and Other Species Associated with Human Habitations, with Special Reference to the Influence of

Temperature and Humidity at Various Periods of the Life History of the Insect', *The Journal of Hygiene*, 13 (1914), 447–654.

Campbell, James M. and R. Mostyn, *Report of the Bombay Plague Committee, Appointed by Government Resolution No. 1204/720P, on the Plague in Bombay, for the Period Extending from the 1st July 1897 to the 30th April 1898* (Bombay: Times of India Steam Press, 1898).

Chandavarkar, Rajnarayan, 'Plague Panic and Epidemic Politics in India, 1896–1914', in: T. O. Ranger and Paul Slack (eds.), *Epidemics and Ideas: Essays on the Historical Perception of Pestilence* (Cambridge, UK: Cambridge University Press, 1992).

Delbourgo, James and Staffan Müller-Wille, 'Introduction', *Isis*, 103, 4 (2012), 710–715: https://doi.org/10.1086/669045.

Echenberg, Myron J., *Plague Ports: The Global Urban Impact of Bubonic Plague, 1894–1901* (New York: New York University Press, 2007).

Edney, Matthew H., *Mapping an Empire: The Geographical Construction of British India, 1765–1843* (Chicago: University of Chicago Press, 1997).

Evans, Nicholas H. A., 'Blaming the Rat? Accounting for Plague in Colonial Indian Medicine', *Medicine Anthropology Theory*, forthcoming.

Fraser, T. R. (ed.), *Indian Plague Commission, 1898–1899. Report of the Indian Plague Commission with Appendices and Summary, Vol. V* (India, Office of the Superintendent of Government Print, 1900).

Gable, Eric, 'Bad Copies: The Colonial Aesthetic and the Manjaco-Portuguese Encounter', in: Deborah D. Kaspin and Paul Stuart Landau (eds.), *Images and Empires: Visuality in Colonial and Postcolonial Africa* (Berkeley: University of California Press, 2002), 294–319.

Gatacre, W. F., *Report on the Bubonic Plague in Bombay, 1896–1897, with Plans* (Bombay: Times of India, 1897).

Gloster, T. H. and F. N. White, 'LXXXIII. Epidemiological Observations in the United Provinces of Agra and Oudh, 1911–1912', *The Journal of Hygiene*, 15 (1917), 793–880.

Hankin, E. H., 'On the Epidemiology of Plague', *The Journal of Hygiene*, 5, 1 (1905), 48–83.

Harley, J. B., 'Deconstructing the Map', *Cartographica*, 26, 2 (1989), 1–20.

Harley, J. B., 'Historical Geography and the Cartographic Illusion', *Journal of Historical Geography*, 15, 1 (1989), 80–91.

Harrison, Mark, 'A Question of Locality: The Identity of Cholera in British India, 1860–1890', in: David Arnold (ed.), *Warm Climates and Western Medicine: The Emergence of Tropical Medicine, 1500–1900* (Amsterdam: Rodopi, 1996), 133–159.

Heinrich, Larissa, *The Afterlife of Images: Translating the Pathological Body between China and the West* (Durham: Duke University Press, 2008).

Hull, Matthew S., *Government of Paper: The Materiality of Bureaucracy in Urban Pakistan* (Berkeley: University of California Press, 2012).

Kidambi, Prashant, '"An Infection of Locality": Plague, Pathogenesis and the Poor in Bombay, c. 1896–1905', *Urban History*, 31, 2 (2004), 249–267.

Kidambi, Prashant, *The Making of an Indian Metropolis: Colonial Governance and Public Culture in Bombay, 1890–1920* (Aldershot: Ashgate, 2007).

Koch, Tom, *Disease Maps: Epidemics on the Ground* (Chicago: University of Chicago Press, 2011).

Koch, Tom, 'Knowing Its Place: Mapping as Medical Investigation', *The Lancet*, 379, 9819 (2012), 887–888: https://doi.org/10.1016/S0140-6736(12)60383-3.

Kunhardt, J. C. and J. Taylor, 'LXXII. Epidemiological Observations in Madras Presidency', *The Journal of Hygiene*, 14 (1915), 683–751.

Lynteris, Christos, 'A "Suitable Soil": Plague's Urban Breeding Grounds at the Dawn of the Third Pandemic', *Medical History*, 61, 3 (2017), 343–357: https://doi.org/10.1017/mdh.2017.32.

Lynteris, Christos, *Ethnographic Plague: Configuring Disease on the Chinese-Russian Frontier* (London: Palgrave Macmillan, 2016).

McLeod, K. S., 'Our Sense of Snow: The Myth of John Snow in Medical Geography', *Social Science & Medicine*, 50, 7–8 (2000), 923–935.

Mohr, James C., *Plague and Fire: Battling Black Death and the 1900 Burning of Honolulu's Chinatown* (Oxford: Oxford University Press, 2006).

Müller-Wille, Staffan and Isabelle Charmantier, 'Lists as Research Technologies', *Isis*, 103, 4 (2012), 743–752: https://doi.org/10.1086/669048.

Nathan, Robert, *The Plague in India, 1896, 1897* (Simla: Government Central Printing Office, 1898).

Numbers, Ronald L., 'Medical Science before Scientific Medicine: Reflections on the History of Medical Geography', *Medical History*, 44, S20 (2000), 217–220.

Peckham, Robert, 'Matshed Laboratory: Colonies, Cultures, and Bacteriology', in: Robert Peckham and David Pomfret, *Imperial Contagions: Medicine, Hygiene, and Cultures of Planning in Asia* (Hong Kong: Hong Kong University Press, 2013), 123–147.

Proctor, Robert and Londa Schiebinger (eds.), *Agnotology: The Making and Unmaking of Ignorance* (Stanford: Stanford University Press, 2008).

Ryan, James R., *Picturing Empire: Photography and the Visualization of the British Empire* (Chicago: University of Chicago Press, 1998).

Samimian-Darash, Limor and Paul Rabinow (eds.), *Modes of Uncertainty: Anthropological Cases* (Chicago: The University of Chicago Press, 2015).

Sarkar, Aditya, 'The Tie That Snapped: Bubonic Plague and Mill Labour in Bombay, 1896–1898', *International Review of Social History*, 59, 02 (2014), 181–214: https://doi.org/10.1017/S0020859014000157.

Sennett, Richard, *Flesh and Stone: The Body and the City in Western Civilization* (London: Faber and Faber, 1994).

Sutphen, Mary P., 'Not What, but Where: Bubonic Plague and the Reception of Germ Theories in Hong Kong and Calcutta, 1894–1897', *Journal of the History of Medicine and Allied Sciences*, 52, 1 (1997), 81–113.

Taussig, Michael, *Mimesis and Alterity: A Particular History of the Senses* (Abingdon: Routledge, 1993).

Taussig, Michael, *Shamanism, Colonialism, and the Wild Man: A Study in Terror and Healing* (Chicago: University of Chicago Press, 1991).

Tucker, E. F. Gordon, *The Management of a Plague Epidemic and the Principles on Which It Should Be Based* (Calcutta: Thacker, Spink & Co., 1906).

Worboys, Michael, *Spreading Germs: Disease Theories and Medical Practice in Britain, 1865–1900* (Cambridge, UK: Cambridge University Press, 2000).

# 6

# 'A SOURCE OF SICKNESS'

## Photographic mapping of the plague in Honolulu in 1900[1]

*Lukas Engelmann*

## Introduction

Frank Davey, a successful but not very well-known photographer of the late nineteenth century, arrived in Hawaii on the steamship 'Australia' on 5 January 1897 to set up a studio in Honolulu.[2] Davey, born and raised in the UK, had worked in Paris, New York, and San Francisco, and set out to capture everyday life in Hawaii, its landscapes and royalty. For nearly ten years, the 'photographer extraordinaire' produced a large archive of sometimes all-too-exotic portraits of Hawaiian kings, indigenous youth and even the odd surfer.[3] The 'mid-pacific metropolis', as Hawaii is called in one of the many celebratory monographs to which Davey contributed a handful of photographs, was at that time emerging as a modern capital at the crossroads of Pacific sea traffic.[4] Recently annexed to the United States of America, the island remained committed to monarchic traditions and indigenous life. Davey's artful portraits focused largely on the latter, assembling and contributing to the picture of an exotic, remote, and melancholic island. The question of epidemics was a long way from his mind and absent from his oeuvre.

Protection against epidemics had become a constant concern in nineteenth-century Hawaii.[5] Vulnerable to diseases from all around the world, the island established its first Board of Health on 13 December 1850, on the orders of King Kamehameha III. A heightened sense of vigilance concerning 'pestilent diseases' carried from Asia and Europe could not halt the epidemics of smallpox in 1851 and 1861. There had been large-scale improvements in sanitation, and new regulations had been put in place. These, however, failed to prevent a cholera outbreak in 1894, and on 12 December 1899, the first case of bubonic plague on the Island was announced to the public.[6]

As soon as the first cases appeared in Honolulu's Chinatown, the Board of Health imposed a quarantine, halted sea traffic, set up a plague hospital, and ordered corpses infected with the disease to be cremated for local containment of the outbreak.[7] To those in charge, the bacteriological cause of the epidemic was undisputed. Yet, the exact form of the bacterium, its vector, the circumstances of its distribution, the mechanics of infection, and conditions of its preservation remained worryingly unclear. Uncertainty about the epidemic's spread was met with political pressure. The economic burden of quarantine led the Board of Health to adopt a set of drastic measures, culminating in the systematic burning of every wooden structure even vaguely associated with plague. This led eventually to the spectacular burning of Honolulu's Chinatown on 20 January 1900, leaving 4,000 homeless, turning the story of the epidemic on the island state into a memory of *Plague and Fire*.[8]

In this emerging crisis, it was the unlikely figure of Davey who – among others – left a visual record of the dramatic fire around Kaumakapili Church.[9] His camera captured the fire brigades, the flames bursting into the church and the apocalyptic landscapes of the scorched territory that used to be Chinatown. But by the time of the fire, his photographic expertise had already been involved in the concerted efforts to drive plague out of Honolulu. Over the course of two weeks, Davey had been commissioned by the Board of Health and had made almost 300 photographs of empty streets, unoccupied houses, outbuildings, and yards affected or even tinged with the suggestion of plague.[10] Davey's series of photographs speaks to us as a meticulous documentation of the space in Honolulu, in which plague occurred, and of the built environment, in which it flourished. Before the sanitary razing of the city spiralled out of control on 20 January, Davey had produced an exhaustive photographic archive of Honolulu's Chinatown, leaving a detailed record of plague's visitations to the city's streets and homes. The images offer an unusual angle, both in the historical narrative of medical photography and the historiography of the third plague pandemic. This chapter draws out the unexpected collaboration between Honolulu's Board of Health and a celebrity photographer to create a photographic record, which proved integral to the strategies employed in containing the epidemic and preventing its return.

Davey's pictures compare well to photographs documenting the plague in other urban centres at the turn of the century. Archives of plague in Hong Kong since 1894, in Oporto in Portugal (1899), Sydney in Australia (1900), and San Francisco in the USA (1900) contain similar series of photographs of inconspicuous street scenes, only indirectly related to the dreaded epidemic, void of people, patients, official personnel, or any measurements.[11] Each album was ordered by, and produced for a local Board of Health; the pictures share an aesthetic of the urban environment, raising concern over the sanitary and hygienic conditions of plague. To the historian, the photographic albums indicate an increased attention to plague's ecology: the structure, shape, and condition of houses, rather than people, that were struck or put 'at risk' by plague. The bacteriological cause or its gruesome manifestation in patients had no place here. For a good part, the photographs are so inconspicuous that their only association with the plague pandemic is to be found in their archival provenance or their metadata.

Other photographic archives of the third plague pandemic exist, which capture sanitary measures, such as fumigation of suspected vectors like rats, gerbils, and marmots, or the effects of plague in patients, photographed in hospitals or quarantine zones. These scenes of epidemic drama captivated the public around the world at the time. While these perspectives seem to fit into established narratives of plague as an epidemic of filth, of rats, and of poverty, Davey's photographic mapping points in a different direction and challenges the historical framework of visual representations of the disease. The question that therefore arises is, what did the neutral and unspectacular recording of plague's environment in urban settings achieve and what had motivated its production in the first place? The case of Honolulu helps us to understand how the production of these photographic records became integral to sanitary campaigns; in what way it became crucial for medical investigation; and whether this photographic practice's popularity with the Board of Health can be best understood through the lens of a threatened hygienic modernity, a standard of hygiene which was deemed to have failed with the return of a centuries-old epidemic.[12]

In Honolulu, the arrival of plague at the end of 1899 was perceived as a failure of modern sanitary standards. The local Board of Health had installed a series of elements to prepare for the eventual arrival of the dreaded disease, but expected to be largely spared from an outbreak of the epidemic, which was not predicted to take hold on any of the islands, and least of all in Honolulu itself.[13] Plague's arrival and outbreak sparked a renewed interest in the particular conditions that enabled plague to be distributed despite the Board's assumed preparedness.[14] Photographic mapping may have contributed to the abstracting capacities of medical geography, supporting an analysis of the epidemic through its configuration and constellation 'on the ground'.[15] But, crucially, it also provided a spatial approach to the epidemic outbreak beyond cartography. Taking on the perspective of a street-level gaze, these photographs enriched any view from above into a series of discrete representations of intimate, local spaces. Each photograph of the built urban landscape extended the cartographic view from a two-dimensional abstraction to take shape as concrete buildings, situations and settings, providing epidemiological portraits of plague's milieu.

Davey's photographic rendering of the plague district merits three historical considerations. First, as other contributions to this volume demonstrate, the photographic configuration of bubonic plague is implicated in the epidemic's medical and scientific conceptualisation. Despite a largely agreed-upon bacteriological agent, the encounter with outbreaks around the globe was not resolved by a laboratory revolution but required a large set of practices in which conflicting and contradicting concepts of disease transmission, contagion and ecology were considered and applied.[16] Plague's bacteriological definition in 1894 did not radically transform it into a laboratory disease but rather turned the arrival of the 'historical disease' in the Americas into a showcase of competing and contradicting medical practices.[17]

Second, embedded in medical and sanitary practices, Davey's photographic archive radically changes the stock history of medical photography. While historiography has mostly been concerned with the clinical and microscopic applications of photography in medicine, Davey's archive adds another layer to the medical incorporation of this technology and paves the way to a history of epidemiological photography, integrating recent contributions to the field.[18]

Third, plague in Honolulu reframed another cornerstone of the early days of the American Public Health system: its racial divide. When the plague reached San Francisco a couple of weeks after Honolulu, it was accompanied by the reiteration of epidemiological and medical reasoning seeking a probable cause for the outbreak with Chinese and Japanese settlers in the city.[19] China was perceived as the geographic origin of the pandemic and 'Chinatown' was seen as the epidemic's local 'breeding ground'. The dwellings were seen as a receptive ecology and a contagious space, accommodating the epidemic as much as posing a risk to the wealthy and predominantly white quarters of the greater city.[20] As Nayan Shah points out, the history of epidemics and Chinese settlement in nineteenth-century USA can rarely be told as separate stories.[21] Furthermore, Shah draws attention to repeated efforts of mapping-out Chinatown as a suspicious space, identified and problematised as the insanitary seedbed of epidemic diseases across the American West. Similar frameworks account for Honolulu, where the begin of the outbreak in Chinatown spiked comparable assumptions and accusations. Despite the fact that the majority of Chinatown's inhabitants had been Japanese workers at the time, prejudice and stereotypes about Chinese customs governed much of the public as well as professional perception of plague in Honolulu.

The photographic mapping of the plague outbreak in Honolulu presents an exemplary case for the complex aetiology that was attributed to the epidemic at the time of its arrival in Honolulu. Set in the wider context of the archive of photographed plague spaces, Davey's photographs expand our appreciation for the breadth of the history of medical photography. This chapter argues that the photographs share with the Board of Health's most dramatic measure – the burning of plague structures – not only a historical connection but moreover a particular sanitary capacity, which condemns the accused building to be a material and expendable embodiment of disease.

## 'A source of filth and a cause of sickness'

In Honolulu preparations for possible outbreaks of plague had been in place since 1898. As part of the Federal Government of the USA, the Marine Hospital Service appointed Duncan A. Carmichael as the first superintendent to oversee operations on the island long before its official annexation to the USA. Carmichael agreed with the Board of Health that the general direction of public health would be based on sound bacteriology.[22]

Dr Walter Hoffmann, Honolulu's chief-bacteriologist, was called immediately when the symptoms of a twenty-two-year-old Chinese bookkeeper, You Chong, who had died on 12 December 1899, seemed to bring the dreaded message that plague had arrived in Honolulu. Hoffmann's microscopic analysis could only confirm what five doctors' clinical expertise had already diagnosed as plague. New reports of patients in Chinatown arrived on the same day, and the Board of Health called an emergency meeting. As James C. Mohr points out, the Board of Health, led by three eminent physicians, then went on to declare a state of emergency on the same day.[23] The Council of State relinquished absolute control over the entire island, which they handed to the Board of Health for as long as the epidemic persisted. With the civilian government of Hawaii suspended, 'three physicians found themselves holding absolute dictatorial authority over all aspects of everyday life in Hawaii'.[24] In the following months, Hawaii was under the governance of a medical body, which turned sanitary regimes, hygienic control and epidemic containment into guiding principles.

The first measures to be imposed were a rigorous quarantine applied to Chinatown, a travel ban, disinfection of premises where plague had been verified or suspected, removal of all ships from the dock, the closure of all business in the harbour and development of water filtration plants, garbage crematoria, and a costly extension of the sewer system.[25] Guided by volunteer brigades, Chinatown was repeatedly and regularly inspected, vigorously surveyed and the epidemic's spread did indeed slow down. According to Lana Iwamoto, the Board of Health's held a strong belief that '[P]lague lives and breeds in filth and when it got into Chinatown, it found its natural habitat'.[26] Chinatown was perceived to be both the harbour and the target of the epidemic. The social dynamic associated with this district, its built environment, its everyday life, contributed to the already racist projection of the 'Yellow Peril' enjoying an alleged natural affiliation to filth, stench and disease.[27]

On 19 December, the quarantine was lifted, as no new cases had been reported for several days. This was premature. The epidemic returned in full-swing on 24 December with nine new cases and twelve more appeared within the next nineteen days, leading to a total of eleven new fatalities. The Board was coerced to undertake drastic measures without any certainty about their efficacy. The question remained: how to locate the bacterium, how to stop it from transmitting from human to human, from animals to humans, from soil to humans, and how, ultimately, it could be eradicated.

A leaflet, distributed to the public of Honolulu on 26 December, suggested measures to be adopted against bubonic plague. The wording reveals the complexity of the ways in which plague was perceived, countered, and thought to be containable. 'Plague germs', the leaflet states, 'flourish in filth, in garbage, and in damp, dark or foul places. Sunlight and pure air are destroyers of plague germs'. Keeping clean, regular washing, keeping scratches and cuts covered, eating fresh and cooked food, were among the suggested precautions. Furthermore, the inguinal buboes located at the lower extremities suggested to the Board of Health that the infection had stemmed from the ground and were harboured in the soil. Bringing scientific weight to this claim, Kitasato was cited as a celebrated plague specialist of the time. Furthermore, the destruction of rats and other vermin was considered crucial and cultural customs such as walking barefoot were considered high risk.[28]

But these measures were not enough. Mohr argues that concern over the safety of white Americans in Hawaii increased pressure on the Board to adopt more drastic strategies. Based on a report of the Sanitary Commission from 29 December that described Chinatown as a 'horribly congested district' in 'a wretched sanitary condition', where fresh meat was exposed within feet of cesspools, where lice and cockroaches were everywhere, and 'shanties, priories, stables, and chicken coops, closely crowded together', only one solution seemed feasible to the Board: to burn every plague-affected structure.[29]

Contrary to common belief, destroying plague's breeding grounds with fire was not a common practice before the third plague pandemic. While the famous Great Fire of London broke out after the 1665 Great Plague, fire might have been used in a number of outbreaks during the nineteenth century, but the outbreak of plague in Hong Kong just five years earlier counts as one of the first documented cases in which fire was considered to be an effective method against plague and its bacterial agent.[30] Fire, many experts around the globe argued, provided the only appropriate measure to destroy wherever 'plague germs' might find accommodation, destroying the agent in its habitat regardless of its character. Still assumed to have been a last resort, fire also provided ultimate security; scorched earth promised a lasting effect against plague.

When the Board of Health in Honolulu decided on 31 December that every built structure associated with the plague within the confines of Chinatown would be burnt, this brought together two aims. Chinatown had become a site of concern to urban planners and white landowners, as rising land prices and the spread of Honolulu seemed to have been held back within these quarters. As Mohr has pointed out, burning most of the wooden structures, which were mostly owned by white elites, did indeed increase the overall land value. The destruction of existing structures were seen as economically beneficial rather than bringing about loss and promised a radical transformation of the urban environment of Honolulu.[31] Furthermore, as Dr Emerson reported to the Board at the time, 'much of the bad conditions in Chinatown were due to faulty construction of buildings', which made sanitary improvements impossible. Large-scale destruction was seen as the only feasible option.[32]

Despite the Board's quasi-dictatorial power, the burning of property, homes, and wooden structures was perceived as a controversial measure, sparking criticism, protest, and even riots. To prevent these reactions, the Board decided to implement a protocol that would strengthen the sanitary authority of the *de facto* government by framing the affected buildings as medical problems, as immediate public health risks. As Mr Cooper, Attorney General and acting President of the Board of Health had undertaken an inspection of block 10 in Chinatown, he and accompanying surveyors 'recommended condemning the entire lot of structures excepting five buildings'.[33] As the minutes reveal, Board members were at the same time cautious regarding the legal and economic implications of planned destructions:

there were two ways of going about it. The legal way was to serve notice on owners and occupants for abatement of nuisances giving them time to do it in, the other way was to go in and destroy the unsanitary structures leaving the matter of damages to be settled later.[34]

Choosing the second option, the Board members were eager to keep legal ramifications as limited as possible and approached the burnings through a series of measures. After a patient had been diagnosed, inspectors would investigate the houses and premises related to plague cases, a report would then be submitted to the Board, which determined the fate of the structure before an independent appraisal committee was sent out to evaluate the economic worth of the structures to be destroyed. From 30 December onwards, the Minutes of the Board begin to contain the repeated and largely formalised ruling with which houses were condemned for burning. From here onwards, almost every daily meeting ended in a similar verdict for different buildings across Chinatown. While frequent attempts were made to identify only those houses in which actual cases occurred, Board members expressed their concern of appearing too cautious in 'not adopting drastic measures'.[35] In the same meeting on 30 December, on the initiative of Dr Smith, it was resolved that the entire Block 10 had to be 'destroyed by fire' (Figure 6.1).[36] On Monday, 1 January, the Board came together to give their verdict on a group of 'infected buildings' on Maunakea Street, adjacent to a building where Wong Hing had recently died of bubonic plague. It was carried that, '[t]he same being declared by this board to be a source of filth and a cause of sickness' should be destroyed by fire.[37] Block 5 was condemned on 2 January and the entirety of Chinatown was declared an infected district on 5 January.[38]

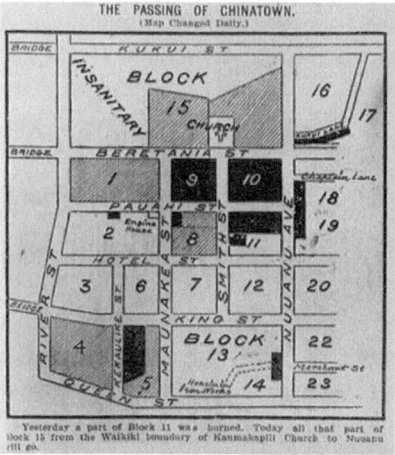

**FIGURE 6.1**   Map of 'The Passing of Chinatown' from early January 1900 detailing the systematic destruction of Chinatown by fire. Hawaii State Archives Digital Collection, PP-19-3-028. With courtesy of the Hawaii State Archives

The Board carried out a kind of diagnostic practice on the houses, building and stretches of land which were declared 'deleterious to the public health'.[39]

Davey and his photographs played a crucial role in the procedures, which led up to the Board's ability to arrive at these verdicts. His photographs paved the way for appropriately appraised cases, leaving visual records of the buildings to be destroyed. They provided a layer of security to the Board and its controversial actions as they were indeed used in the aftermath of the epidemic as evidence in case files, marked with numbers to be referenced to a map.[40]

On the other hand, Davey's series of photographed plague houses suggests an involvement of photographs in the process of transforming a building into a health risk, of making non-human, non-sentient elements of the urban environment of Honolulu sources of filth and sickness. Davey's photographic mapping of plague in Chinatown appears to have bolstered the reasoning of public health and epidemiology beyond the capacities of clinical medicine and laboratory science.

## Photographic portraits of plague houses

One such photograph taken by Frank Davey shows a local saloon, the Beehive (Figure 6.2). The photograph bears the signature style, which he developed in his break-away from the royal and romantic portraits, to focus on inanimate environments. The photograph captured an apparently inconspicuous street scene. There are buildings, wooden structures, a couple of people seem accidentally to populate the side of the frame. Indisputably the photograph centres on the saloon itself. Davey's name and a number are written on the front, while on the back another number is engraved and a series of pencil notes indicate that this image is part of a set of archival framings of bubonic plague, taken in January 1900. The photograph outside its archival setting hardly resembles a visual iconography typically associated with bubonic plague. It does not show symptoms; it does not picture bodily remains of a deadly epidemic; there are no activities of disinfection, fumigation, or quarantine. It just shows one of many buildings, understood to be a danger to public health, a diagnosis which is nowhere evident in the image itself, and only derives from the photograph.

On 10 January 1900, the Minutes of the Board read:

> It was unanimously resolved that the premises known as the Bee Hive Saloon on Nuuanu Street, the same having been inspected by this Board are in the opinion of this Board insanitary, a source of filth and a cause of sickness, and are incapable of being rendered sanitary by fumigation or other means, and that it is necessary for the public health and safety that the buildings on the same should be destroyed by fire.[41]

This same phrasing was applied to a further thirty-five properties at that same meeting. Destruction was to be carried out as soon as possible. Davey's photographs of these and many more buildings (Figure 6.3) resembled the serial diagnostic

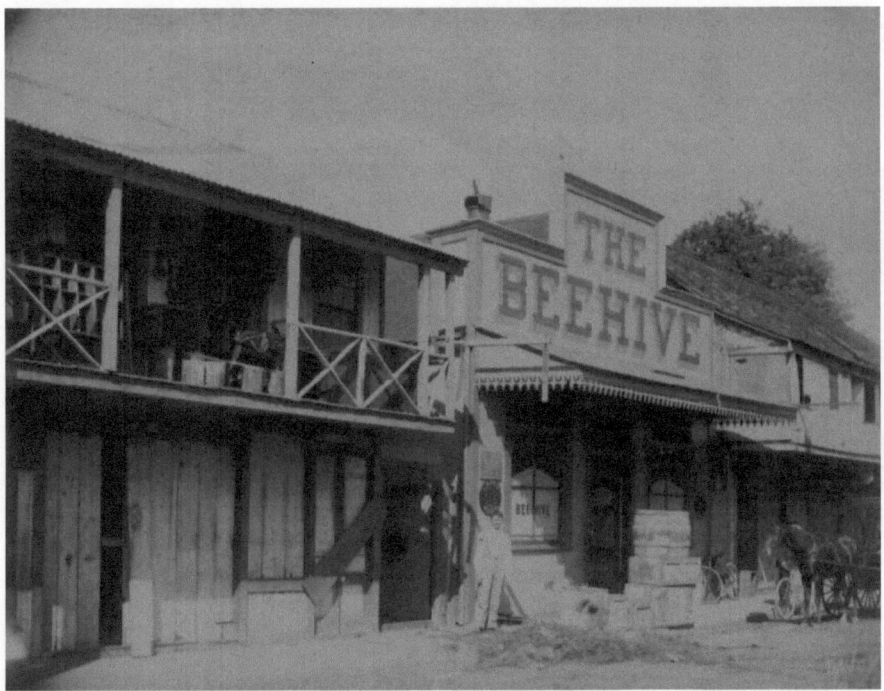

**FIGURE 6.2**    Photograph by Frank Davey for the Honolulu Board of Health depicting the 'Beehive' saloon on Nuuanu Street. Taken in early January 1900, 'during the Bubonic Plague' (handwritten note on back), Hawaii State Archives Digital Collection, PP-17-11-022-00001. With courtesy of the Hawaii State Archives

effort carried out on a large number of houses in Chinatown. The images of the Hawaiian album show streets, alleys, houses, and huts in different shapes and constitutions; they sometimes include furniture put out on the streets for fumigation. Every now and then we see people, maybe inhabitants, captured by chance in the backgrounds, and other personnel, soldiers, or members of official services in the foreground. But patients and their actions, catastrophic events and their effects are not the determining focus of the photographs. On the contrary, the protagonists haunting these images are the buildings and streets, situations, and configurations of space and locality. Davey's at first-glance inconspicuous photographs show us places which, if deprived of their archival rendering as visual representations of the plague, share a characteristic feature of being unremarkable, of picturing an absence of purpose.

The global archive of plague photography at the turn of the century reflects the coexistence of different kinds of photographic archives.[42] In contrast to the longstanding visual history of plague, the third plague pandemic was rarely pictured through representations of bodily symptoms, scenes of social unrest, but

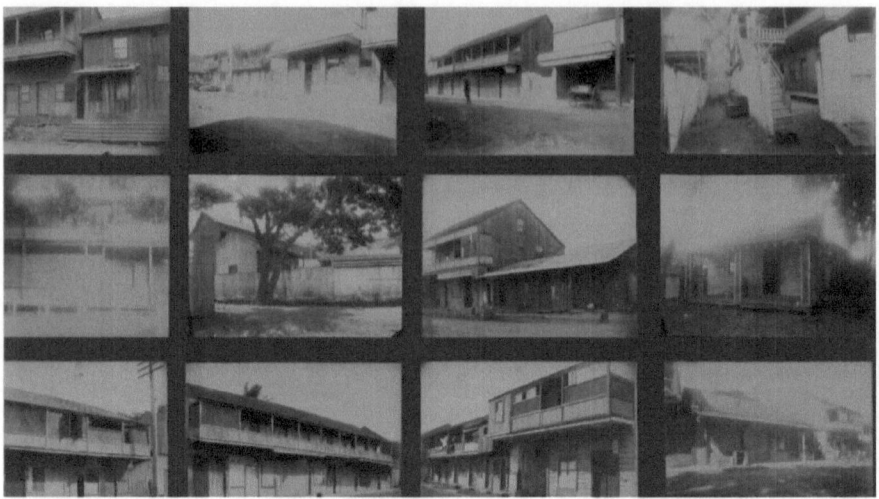

**FIGURE 6.3**   Twelve photographs from Frank Davey's series for the Honolulu Board of Health, taken in early January 1900. Hawaii State Archives Digital Collection, various call numbers. Courtesy of the Hawaii State Archives

photographs were mostly used to capture governmental and medical measures to combat the epidemic's spread: fumigation of clothes and furniture, disinfection of areas, grounds, and personal belongings, demolition of buildings and structures, and countless pictures displaying the purifying effects of fire, not to mention rat-trapping, rat-examinations, and pictures of rat burrows and their breeding grounds. Against this backdrop, the photographic mapping of Honolulu – and equally San Francisco, Sydney, and Oporto – share a remarkable lack of significant references regarding measures, actions, events, or catastrophes. This emptiness, combined with the sheer volume of pictures taken, provides an opportunity to rediscover a different historic way of seeing, understanding, and containing plague. Davey's photographs stand out precisely because of their lack of expected significant icons, symbols, and references, an expectation which gives valuable information to the historian regarding what we have learnt to think what plague would or should look like.

Words written in pencil on the back of many of Davey's photographs indicate that the pictures were taken explicitly for the Board of Health. But is the production of the album, therefore, to be assumed to have been guided by strict medical considerations? Medical photography has traditionally been understood to have derived from a visual tradition of framing pathological anatomy through illustrations or wax moulage.[43] As an effort to further establish medicine as guided by scientific principles, the celebrated mechanical objectivity of photography lent both authority and popularity to the medico-photographic profession in Europe and the USA.[44] The nineteenth century saw a surge of photographs taken which obsessed over unusual pathological sightings, monstrous deformations and spectacular diseases.[45] Part documentation, part freak-show, the photographs tended to be concerned with the exceptions and not the rules. But instead of deformed bodies, marked with the spectacular skin eruptions of bubonic plague – buboes – Davey's archive offers rows of pictures of humble houses in an unremarkable urban environment. The questions which remain are: what drove the Board of Health to order these street photographs to be taken? Why was Davey chosen with his flair for taking portraits of glamour and exoticism? And what purpose did the photographs serve to understand, contain and finally to burn out plague?

In the second half of the nineteenth century, photography had been used in a variety of experimental fashions for medical and physiological interrogations. Photography was applied to the study of movements.[46] The effects of being photographed on patients with mental illness has been studied by Charcot in Paris' Salpêtrière, and photography had already developed a position beyond classic portraiture of patients and their symptoms.[47] As Jeanne Haffner has recently shown, photography was also applied to the study of phenomena whose visualisation required new technologies and experimental procedures: to rethink the social relations of population in urban environments, to establish a science of the social space, and to create a discourse about the urban areas, the camera claimed a bird's eye view to establish a view from above.[48] But Davey's eye-level rather than bird's eye view perspective, and the photographic practices deployed in Hawaii, mirror a new way of seeing plague outbreaks: not generalised and impersonal, but assumed to be linked to the particular hygiene of individual houses, of street corners and small but racially framed communities. The urban spaces of Sydney or Porto and Honolulu, which were assumed to have been sanitarily robust, were exposed in their vulnerability. The production of the photographic record of plague's urban appearances, the epidemic's built 'cases', created a visibility in which the reason for a failing hygienic standard as much as the disease itself was always implied, but hardly ever seen.

## Photographic mapping of plague

Mapping the urban landscape of plague reinvented the photographic album as an instrument of interrogation and surveillance. As a record of the conditions, the appearances and the structures in which plague occurred, the album presents a case file, in which not only single houses, but the social space of Chinatown, and accordingly the racial stereotypes attached to it, were rendered into targets of destruction. Photography also allowed the visualisation of the epidemic's ambiguous and elusive nature. The bacteriological agent did not provide an understanding immediately allowing inspectors to curb its distribution or to destroy the conditions of its survival: where and how plague appeared and thrived remained at the time of the Honolulu outbreak an open-ended question, accommodated best in the equally open-ended faculty of photographic mapping.

As such, Davey's visual practice in the case of Honolulu, is perhaps best resembled in the early modern efforts of the urban mapping of plague. Nicholas Eckstein describes the case of Florence, where plague had been met with a rigorous public health response; a mapping of the urban environment of plague achieved through observations and their systematic recordings, the '*relazioni*'.[49] Implicated in the policy of mapping and tracking the poor accused of having caused plague, 'eye-level mapping' could establish an understanding of the situation in which plague was thriving. The bird's eye view and its abstracted equivalent – the cartographic map – 'presents the urban space and the city as a theoretical representation of itself, a flattened optical artefact drained of the contingency, variety and incompleteness that are essential qualities of everyday life', as Eckstein reminds us.[50] But the details, the particularity, the variety, and the irreducibility of urban life appeared in the descriptions of the '*Visitatori*', who experienced urban life on foot, to apprehend in full the scope of the emergency of plague. In 1630 Florence, the proximity of tightly knit neighbourhoods was associated with corruption, miasmatic odours, and filth as the cause of plague.[51]

Translated and carefully compared to the turn-of-the-century mapping of Chinatown, these records of the social life of plague were turned into a racialised narrative. As Shah has shown for the case of plague in Chinatown in San Francisco, public health was organised along the lines of territorial divisions, which was reflected in the contrast between a 'Chinese race' and the 'American people'.[52] The space of Chinatown was fundamental to the construction of Chinese difference and white norms. Remarkably close to Eckstein's description of Florence's aristocratic perception of the poor quarters, Honolulu's Chinese and Japanese settlements were perceived as a strenuous living environment, in which density characterised a lifestyle assumed to breed filth, odour and corruption as the perfect conditions for diseases like bubonic plague.

The appearance of plague in Honolulu offered those in charge a seemingly legitimate excuse to shape a health policy directed against the populations living in Chinatown, exercised through recording, analysing and mapping of its urban environment.[53] Where Shah emphasises the panoptical effect of maps as instruments of political power, crafting oversight, order, and spatial coordinates in a space perceived as opaque, dense and threatening to a public health concerned with white-population, the plague album of Honolulu suggests an advanced application of mapping. Traditional maps, the geographer Harley reminds us, tend 'to "desocialise" the territory they represent, fostering the notion of a socially empty space'.[54] Abstracting the landscape and its particularities in a diagrammatic representation, a map delivered an empty space, void of social life and therefore lacking instant utility to act upon plague's appearance in Honolulu.

A photographic mapping of buildings provided something new and valuable to the eyes of the Honolulu Board of Health. Plague houses were neither spectacular nor could their visual appearance be identified as symptomatic of plague. Photography was not applied here to capture significant details about the conditions of the distribution of the 'plague germ', nor did it capture characteristic details of insanitary conditions. The album was not produced with an interest in further understanding and abstracting the nature of plague, but to enable and to justify a sanitary policy. The burning of privately owned houses required an official verdict, rendering the house a nuisance for public health, which in turn led photographs to be taken with the purpose of underlining the house's dangerous significance in a situation of epidemic crisis.

Contrary to many readings of medical photography in the nineteenth century, this practice did not increase the scientific merit of the Board of Health.[55] Moreover, the pictures of the houses did not contain any information to contribute further to an analytical and abstracting understanding of what plague was. Nor did they deliver signs of infestation or traces of death and despair. Photography was not an instrument of medical interrogation but was instead used to visually frame inconspicuous houses as objects of epidemiological significance.

Photographic mapping could, therefore, be understood as the medical portraiture of an epidemic's ecology, capturing the disease on the ground by means of mapping a sequence of houses and places, bound together by suspicions and assumed appearances and possible instances of the same disease. Davey's album presents a series of seemingly unconnected peculiarities that make up the infected plague-ridden space. As medical photography, commissioned by the Board of Health to bolster the case of diagnosing houses as 'sources of filth and causes of sickness', the sequence of pictures did not contribute to a refined bacteriological understanding of plague, nor did it relocate the epidemic to the laboratory or give grounds for systematic analysis of vectors, such as rats or fleas. The photographs comprise evidence that the Board had to abandon the lure of science for an altogether different approach: If anything, photographic mapping reconfigured a tradition of thinking about diseases in their urban embodiment through spatial coordinates, populated territories, and built environments. In light of Davey's work, the history of medical photography is thus in need of a critical extension beyond clinical, psychiatric, and bacteriological applications to include the larger history of visualising disease in medical geography.

## Medical geography beyond cartography

As a 'medical science before scientific medicine', medical geography had established a unique value to understand specific diseases before the time of the laboratory.[56] Throughout the nineteenth century, plague had found a prominent place in major publications of the thriving field. Perhaps its most characteristic description was given by August Hirsch in his renowned *Handbook of Geographical and Historical Pathology*.[57] Hirsch incorporated a series of aetiological theories and discussed implications of germ theory, the involvement of rodents and rats as well as miasmatic models to form a comprehensive account of plague's relation to space. The assumption of local peculiarities enabled an interpretation of the disease through spatial coordinates, local conditions, and particular structures without arriving at a fixed aetiology.[58] Medical geography found its motives in the interrogation, aggregation and *mapping* of 'local peculiarities', to arrive at what Susan Craddock has described, in the case of San Francisco, as 'spatial pathologies'.[59]

Erwin Ackerknecht has famously argued that medical geography should be understood as an integral element in the genesis of modern disease specificity. Endeavours to combine historical narratives with geographical structures made disease entities graspable precisely through their connection to spaces.[60] The notion of spatial configurations was never understood as a radical contradiction to bacteriological science, but rather seems always to have had an independent status. The map, medical geography's instrument to arrive at two-dimensional representations of disease, has been used since early modern times to deliver abstract accounts, theories, and models of the epidemic's relation to particular spaces.[61]

Tom Koch's extensive writings on the history of medical mapping make a strong case for understanding maps beyond visual representations of spatial situations of diseases. Maps were involved in transforming the individual case and its pathology into a public health event, turning a cluster of single cases into a constellation of spatially located incidences. But maps have also been used throughout history as an instrument to test theories about diseases within spatial boundaries.[62] Maps were not only used to capture diseases in space but to think through the spatial peculiarities to arrive at an improved strategy for containment. This implies an understanding of mapping as a way of *making* arguments. The map was and is a tool to incite visual thinking about diseases in space and thus as 'a method of assemblage in which ideas are constituted'.[63] Koch presents the map as a method of interrogation, as a thinking device, and even as an experimental system to demonstrate that mapping is a process which is at once graphic, numerical, spatial, and theoretical.[64]

Understanding Davey's pictures as spatial reasoning translated into photographic visualisation allows us to contemplate a medical geography beyond cartography. Having moved beyond the limitations of maps, their abstraction and de-populated representations of spatial coordinates, Davey's photographs deliver a series of portraits of places implicated in an epidemic. The representation of the space of plague thereby achieved did not, and was not designed to, shed light on an aetiological solution. The series of photographs rather interrogate plague in its 'local peculiarities' so as to deliver to the Board a way of seeing plague that does not provide aetiological depth but remains on the surface of the epidemic's urban body, visualising the infected structures that harbour the invisible danger.

Photography in the service of medical geography, therefore, provides a mapping of the plague milieu in the city of Honolulu that, as Elizabeth Edwards has pointed out elsewhere, 'awakens a desire to know that which it cannot show'.[65] Photographic mapping falls short in delivering a well-defined model of why plague broke out in the urban environment of Honolulu. Davey's photographs instead show a series of locations associated with plague (in non-specific ways) that 'house' the plague 'germs' while dampening specific questions about aetiology. As such, the application of photographic mapping visually preserves what the burning of Chinatown achieved: rather than elucidating the dilemma, the photographs emphasise indifference to the disease's origin, instead supporting a more general endeavour to purge the suspicious environment of Chinatown from the urban landscape.

## Conclusion

The precise purpose of Davey's photographs for the Board of Health remains subject to speculation. A source which indicates the Board's motives for employing the romantic, some might say unsuitable, photographer for the task of rendering houses into threats of public health remains a missing link. The traces stitched together in this chapter comprise circumstantial evidence rather than a conclusive disclosure. Documents indicate that the photographs were used directly by the Board, by an appraisal commission which suggests an association between the photographs and an accompanying map. The map has not yet been unearthed, and as it may have been drawn on the wall of the Board's office, it may never be discovered.

The annotations on the back of the photographs, the titles on the lids of the boxes and associated digital metadata are what anchors Davey's photographs in their relation to the 1899 plague outbreak. To approach these photographs with anything less than precise attention to their archival provenance is to render them unrecognisable as plague photographs. The way this collection presents itself to the historian thus reflects the circumstance of its production and utilisation at the time of plague in Honolulu. Rather than covering, documenting, and archiving scenes of plague, the act of ordering, taking and preserving the pictures upon orders of the Board of Health is what transforms their content, their architectural subjects, into threatening plague houses, buildings as 'a source of sickness'.

This chapter has addressed a particular photographic practice as a technique of mapping. Photographs taken in the service of public health at the turn of the century have integrated the constructive, thought-provoking faculties of abstraction possible in medical geography. Refusing to pursue the goal of visualising the disease in its aetiological depth, Davey's is a portraiture of the urban plague space. His photographic mapping might not have supported hypotheses about plague's aetiology, nor did they offer conclusions on the material conditions of the bacteria's nesting grounds. But the album enabled and helped to justify drastic measures deemed necessary to contain epidemic threats. Within the history of medical photography, this epidemiological dimension of medical photography has not yet been understood in depth and is in need of further research across different spaces, epidemics and public health contexts.

Located in between heightened uncertainty about plague's mode of transmission and the drastic measure of burning every suspected, affected, and infected structure, both the rhetorical verdict recorded in the 'Minutes' of the Board, as well as the photographs taken by Davey, contributed to the production of diagnostic evidence for the built environment that points beyond the bacteriological laboratory, beyond the clinic and even beyond the geographic map. Davey's portraits drew together a sequence of plague spaces which made up the urban surface of the epidemic threat, and in this way, his practice constituted a form of epidemiological photography.

## Notes

1 Research leading to this chapter was funded by the European Research Council Starting Grant under the European Union's Seventh Framework Programme/ERC grant agreement no. 336564; European Research Council [FP7/2007–2013] for the project Visual Representations of the Third Plague Pandemic (CRASSH, University of Cambridge).
2 'Notes', *The Hawaiian Star*, 5 January 1897, 8.
3 Echenberg, *Plague Ports*, 207.
4 Whitney, *Hawaiian America*.
5 Lee, 'History of Public Health in Hawaii'; Moran, *Colonizing Leprosy*.
6 Eskey, 'Epidemiological Study of Plague in the Hawaiian Islands'; 'Bubonic Plague, Breed of Filth, Here', *The Hawaiian Star*, 12 December 1899, 1.
7 Ikeda, 'A Brief History of Bubonic Plague'; Iwamoto, 'The Plague and Fire of 1899–1900'. On the question of post-mortem contagion see also the contributions to Lynteris/Evan, *Histories of Post-Mortem Contagion*.
8 Mohr, *Plague and Fire*.
9 See for example photograph PP-18-2-026-00001, Hawaii State Archives.
10 Due to the absence of direct documentation, the commission can only be reconstructed through evidence pointing indirectly to Davey having carried out the photographic recordings for the Board of Health, as will be shown further below.
11 For the photographs of Hong Kong' plagued houses, see Peckham, Chapter 4, this volume, for Oporto, see the collection 'Foto Guedes' at Arquivo Histórico Municipal do Porto, F-NV-FG-M-04-0028. For Sydney, see State Library New South Wales' collections on Bubonic Plague, 1900. For San Francisco, see the Williamson Album at San Francisco Public Library (uncatalogued, no call number).
12 Rogaski, *Hygienic Modernity*.
13 Mohr, *Plague and Fire*, 16.
14 On the history and present of the concept of preparedness, see Caduff, *The Pandemic Perhaps*.
15 Koch, *Disease Maps*. Hardy, *Epidemic Streets*.
16 For a systematic take on plague's bacteriology in San Francisco: Engelmann, 'A Plague of Kinyounism'.
17 Cunningham, 'Transforming Plague'; Hardy, 'On the Cusp: Epidemiology and Bacteriology'; Weindling, 'From Infectious to Chronic Diseases'; Lynteris, 'Ethnographic Plague'.
18 Lynteris and Prince, 'Anthropology and Medical Photography'; Gradmann, *Krankheit im Labor*; Haffner, *The View from Above*; Mifflin, 'Visual Archives in Perspective'; Schlich, '"Wichtiger als der Gegenstand selbst"'; Tucker, *Nature Exposed*.
19 Chase, *The Barbary Plague*; Risse, *Plague, Fear, and Politics*.
20 Echenberg, *Plague Ports*, 186.
21 Shah, *Contagious Divides*.
22 Mohr, *Plague and Fire*, 50.
23 The three physicians with the Board of Health were the 'vaccinating officer' Dr Nathaniel B. Emerson, and his two long standing colleagues and friends Dr Francis R. Day and Dr Clifford B. Wood, *Ibid.*, 41 ff.
24 *Ibid.*, 40.
25 Ikeda, 'A Brief History'; Mohr, *Plague and Fire*, 84.
26 Iwamoto, 'The Plague and Fire'. This sentiment about a particular space within the larger pace of the city is matched by contemporaries to plague outbreaks at least since the seventeenth century, see Henderson, Chapter 3, this volume.
27 Frayling, *The Yellow Peril*.
28 Board of Health, Honolulu, *Regulations against Bubonic Plague*, Leaflet, in: Hawaii State Archives, Incoming Letters, Board of Health, 1899–1900.
29 Cited in: Iwamoto, 'The Plague and Fire of 1899–1900', 380.

30 While it was never used in Hong Kong, other sources suggest fire has been used against plague outbreaks in Vetlianka, 1878, in Anzob 1898, and in India after 1896. See contributions of Lynteris and Evans, Chapter 5, this volume.
31 Mohr, *Plague and Fire*, 90. This also resembles similar discussion on real estate speculation and plague demolition in Hong Kong, see Lynteris, Introduction, this volume.
32 Honolulu Board of Health, 'Minutes, January 1 1899–April 31 1900, Volume 8' (1899), 111, State Archive Hawaii, 259.
33 *Ibid.*, 121.
34 *Ibid.*
35 *Ibid.*
36 *Ibid.*, 122.
37 *Ibid.*, 125.
38 *Ibid.*, 127, 131.
39 *Ibid.*, 138.
40 See letter from Ripley, Wilhelm *et al.* on March 20, 1900, referencing numbers to have been marked on 'photographs of the buildings' in regards to the survey and appraisal services undertaken for the Board of Health, in: Hawaii State Archives, Incoming Letters, Board of Health, 1899–1900.
41 Honolulu Board of Health, Minutes, January 1 1899–April 31 1900, Volume 8, 145.
42 Poleykett *et al.*, 'Fragments of Plague'.
43 Donald, 'The History of Medical Illustration'; Schnalke, *Diseases in Wax*.
44 Fox and Lawrence, *Photographing Medicine*; Daston and Galison, 'The Image of Objectivity'; Tucker, *Nature Exposed*; Sheehan, *Doctored*.
45 Burns, *Early Medical Photography in America*; Heinrich, *The Afterlife of Images*.
46 Braun and Whitcombe, 'Marey, Muybridge, and Londe'; Morgan, 'Edward Muybridge and W. S. Playfair'.
47 Didi-Huberman, *Invention of Hysteria*.
48 Haffner, *View from Above*, 7.
49 Eckstein, 'Florence on Foot, 6. See also Henderson, Chapter 3, this volume.
50 *Ibid.*, 12.
51 *Ibid.*, 20.
52 Shah, *Contagious Divides*, 42.
53 *Ibid.*, 17.
54 Harley, 'Maps, Knowledge and Power', 303.
55 Tucker, *Nature Exposed*.
56 Numbers, 'Medical Science before Scientific Medicine, Rupke (ed.), *Medical Geography in Historical Perspective*; Valencius, 'Histories of Medical Geography'.
57 Hirsch, *Handbook of Geographical and Historical Pathology*.
58 *Ibid.*, 521.
59 Craddock, *City of Plagues*, 10.
60 Ackerknecht, *Geschichte und Geographie der wichtigsten Krankheiten*.
61 Jarcho, 'Some Early Italian Epidemiological Maps'.
62 Koch, *Disease Maps*, 2.
63 *Ibid.*, 13.
64 *Ibid.*
65 Edwards, *Raw Histories*, 18.

# References

## Primary sources

*The Hawaiian Star*, Newspaper, Honolulu.
Honolulu Board of Health Minutes, 1 January 1899–April 1900, Vol. 8, Hawaii State Archive.

Incoming Letters, Board of Health, 1899–1900, Hawaii State Archives.
Photographic Collection, Hawaii State Archives.

## Secondary literature

Ackerknecht, Erwin H., *Geschichte und Geographie der wichtigsten Krankheiten* (Stuttgart: Enke, 1963).

Anderson, Warwick, *Colonial Pathologies: American Tropical Medicine, Race, and Hygiene in the Philippines* (Durham, NC: Duke University Press, 2006).

Bashford, Alison, *Imperial Hygiene: A Critical History of Colonialism, Nationalism and Public Health* (Basingstoke: Palgrave Macmillan, 2004).

Braun, Marta and Elizabeth Whitcombe, 'Marey, Muybridge, and Londe', *History of Photography*, 23, 3 (1999), 218–224.

Burns, Stanley B., *Early Medical Photography in America (1839–1883)* (New York: Burns Archive, 1983).

Caduff, Carlo, *The Pandemic Perhaps: Dramatic Events in a Public Culture of Danger* (Oakland: University of California Press, 2015).

Chase, Marilyn, *The Barbary Plague: The Black Death in Victorian San Francisco* (London: Random House Publishing Group, 2004).

Craddock, Susan, *City of Plagues: Disease, Poverty, and Deviance in San Francisco* (Minneapolis: University of Minnesota Press, 2000).

Cunningham, Andrew, 'Transforming Plague: The Laboratory and the Identity of Infectious Disease', in: Andrew Cunningham and Perry Williams (eds.), *The Laboratory Revolution in Medicine* (Cambridge, UK: Cambridge University Press, 1992), 209–244.

Daston, Lorraine and Peter Galison, 'The Image of Objectivity', *Representations*, 40 (1992), 81–128.

Didi-Huberman, Georges, *Invention of Hysteria: Charcot and the Photographic Iconography of the Salpetriere* (Cambridge, MA: MIT Press, 2003).

Donald, Gabriel, 'The History of Medical Illustration', *Journal of Audiovisual Media in Medicine*, 9 (1986), 44–49.

Echenberg, Myron J., *Plague Ports: The Global Urban Impact of Bubonic Plague, 1894–1901* (New York: New York University Press, 2007).

Eckstein, Nicholas A., 'Florence on Foot: An Eye-Level Mapping of the Early Modern City in Time of Plague', *Renaissance Studies*, 30, 2 (2016), 273–297.

Edwards, Elizabeth, *Raw Histories: Photographs, Anthropology and Museums* (London: Bloomsbury Academic, 2001).

Engelmann, Lukas, 'A Plague of Kinyounism, Caricatures of Bacteriology in 1900 San Francisco', *Social History of Medicine*, forthcoming.

Eskey, Clifford Rush, 'Epidemiological Study of Plague in the Hawaiian Islands', *Public Health Reports*, 50, 8 (1934), 255–257.

Fox, Daniel M. and Christopher Lawrence, *Photographing Medicine: Images and Power in Britain and America since 1840* (New York: Greenwood Press, 1988).

Frayling, Christopher, *The Yellow Peril: Dr Fu Manchu & the Rise of Chinaphobia* (London: Thames & Hudson, 2014).

Gradmann, Christoph, *Krankheit im Labor: Robert Koch und die medizinische Bakteriologie* (Göttingen: Wallstein, 2005).

Haffner, Jeanne, *The View from Above: The Science of Social Space* (Cambridge, MA: MIT Press, 2013).

Hardy, Anne, *The Epidemic Streets: Infectious Disease and the Rise of Preventive Medicine, 1856–1900* (Wotton-under-Edge: Clarendon Press, 1993).

Hardy, Anne, 'On the Cusp: Epidemiology and Bacteriology at the Local Government Board, 1890–1905', *Medical History*, 42, 3 (1998), 328–346

Harley, J. B., 'Maps, Knowledge and Power', in: D. Cosgrove and S. Daniels (eds.), *The Iconography of Landscape* (Cambridge, UK: University of Cambridge Press, 1988), 277–312.

Heinrich, Ari Larissa, *The Afterlife of Images: Translating the Pathological Body between China and the West* (Durham, NC: Duke University Press, 2008).

Hirsch, August, *Handbook of Geographical and Historical Pathology* (London: New Sydenham Society, 1883).

Ikeda, James K., 'A Brief History of Bubonic Plague in Hawaii', *Proceedings of the Hawaiian Entomological Society*, 25 (1985), 75–81.

Iwamoto, Lana, 'The Plague and Fire of 1899–1900 in Honolulu', *Hawaii Historical Review*, 2, 8 (1967), 379–394.

Jarcho, Saul, 'Some Early Italian Epidemiological Maps', *Imago Mundi*, 35, 1 (1983), 9–19.

Koch, Tom, *Disease Maps: Epidemics on the Ground* (Chicago: University of Chicago Press, 2011).

Lee, R. K., 'History of Public Health in Hawaii', *Hawaii Medical Journal*, 15, 4 (1956), 331–337.

Lynteris, Christos. *Ethnographic Plague: Configuring Disease on the Chinese–Russian Frontier* (Basingstoke: Palgrave Macmillan, 2016).

Lynteris, Christos and Nicholas H. A. Evans (eds.), *Histories of Post-Mortem Contagion: Infected Corpses and Contested Burials* (Basingstoke: Palgrave Macmillan, 2018).

Lynteris, Christos and Ruth J. Prince, 'Anthropology and Medical Photography: Ethnographic, Critical and Comparative Perspectives', *Visual Anthropology*, 29, 2 (2016), 101–117.

Mifflin, Jeffrey, 'Visual Archives in Perspective: Enlarging on Historical Medical Photographs', *The American Archivist*, 70, 1 (2007), 32–69.

Mohr, James C., *Plague and Fire: Battling Black Death and the 1900 Burning of Honolulu's Chinatown* (New York: Oxford University Press, 2005).

Moran, Michelle Therese, *Colonizing Leprosy: Imperialism and the Politics of Public Health in the United States* (Chapel Hill: University of North Carolina Press, 2007).

Morgan, Jayne, 'Edward Muybridge and W. S. Playfair', *History of Photography*, 23, 3 (1999), 225–231.

Numbers, R. L., 'Medical Science before Scientific Medicine: Reflections on the History of Medical Geography', *Medical History Supplement*, 20 (2000), 217–220.

Poleykett, Branwyn, Lukas Engelmann, and Nicholas H.A. Evans 'Fragments of Plague', *Limn* (2016): http://limn.it/fragments-of-plague, accessed 7 March 2016.

Risse, Guenter B., *Plague, Fear, and Politics in San Francisco's Chinatown* (Baltimore: Johns Hopkins University Press, 2012).

Rogaski, Ruth, *Hygienic Modernity: Meanings of Health and Disease in Treaty-Port China* (Oakland: University of California Press, 2004).

Rupke, Nicolaas A. (ed.), *Medical Geography in Historical Perspective* (London: Wellcome Trust Centre for the History of Medicine at UCL, 2000).

Schlich, Thomas, '"Wichtiger als der Gegenstand selbst" – Die Bedeutung des fotografischen Bildes in der Begründung der bakteriologischen Krankheitsauffassung durch Robert Koch', in: Martin Dinges and Thomas Schlich (eds.), *Neue Wege in der Seuchengeschichte* (Stuttgart: Franz Steiner Verlag, 1995), 143–152.

Schnalke, Thomas, *Diseases in Wax: The History of the Medical Moulage* (Chicago: Quintessence Publications, 1995).

Shah, Nayan, *Contagious Divides: Epidemics and Race in San Francisco's Chinatown* (Oakland, CA: University of California Press, 2001).

Sheehan, Tanya, *Doctored. The Medicine of Photography in Nineteenth-Century America* (University Park: Pennsylvania State University Press, 2011).

Tucker, Jennifer, *Nature Exposed: Photography as Eyewitness in Victorian Science* (Baltimore: Johns Hopkins University Press, 2005).

Weindling, Paul, 'From Infectious to Chronic Diseases: Changing Patterns of Sickness in the Nineteenth and Twentieth Centuries', in: Andrew Wear (ed.), *Medicine in Society; Historical Essays* (Cambridge, UK: Cambridge University Press, 1992), 303–316.

Valencius, C. B., 'Histories of Medical Geography', *Medical History Supplement*, 20 (2000), 3–28.

Whitney, Caspar, *Hawaiian America: Something of Its History, Resources, and Prospects* (New York: Harper & Brothers, 1899).

# 7

# PUBLIC CULTURE AND THE SPECTACLE OF EPIDEMIC DISEASE IN RABAT AND CASABLANCA[1]

*Branwyn Poleykett*

In the aftermath of highly mediatised global events, such as the outbreak of severe acute respiratory syndrome (SARS, 2002–2003) and the 2014 Ebola epidemic in West Africa, contemporary epidemics are often theorised and experienced as spectacular events, consumed by a rapt global audience fascinated by the images of mass death and possibilities of socio-political unravelling. Historians and social scientists have written at length about what Priscilla Wald calls the 'outbreak narrative', the formulaic story of emergence, expansion, and containment whose roots can be found in the epidemiological assumptions of late nineteenth-century urbanism.[2] Outbreak narratives impose the illusion of scientific control on chaotic, complex, and opaque events, shaping them into a coherent and explicable whole.

What has been granted less attention within this work are the representational regimes and material apparatuses that have worked to contain and to suppress the fact of infectious disease. Colonial cities were built to contain the open secret of disease, to materially enclose contagion, and to encode and display their hygienic values via architectural and aesthetic innovation. In the Moroccan cities of Rabat and Casablanca during the French Protectorate, outbreaks of infectious disease were decidedly muted events shrouded in secrecy and characterised by ambiguity. Information about outbreaks of disease were strategically withheld from the public during the world wars and in the period I examine here this information continued to be treated as potentially politically explosive. The archive bears traces, for example, of censored reports with dates and neighbourhoods slashed through and the words 'plague' or 'typhus' replaced with identifying numbers.

Rabat and Casablanca were intensely mediatised cities; relentlessly depicted by artists, photographers, and filmmakers who sought to capture the salvage and curatorial role of French authorities in 'preserving' the antique and picturesque Moroccan presence in the colonial cities, while applying rational planning principles to the shaping of the new quarters, the whole forming and aesthetically pleasing, politically integrated but socially segregated urban unit. The integrative work of Moroccan urbanism founded new genres of writing about urban environments; experimental urbanism, medical geography, and new forms of city-writing and cinematography thrived in colonial North African cities in the first half of the twentieth century in response to the novel representational demands of this singular city space. All of these new genres attempted to grapple with three forms of early twentieth-century urban spectacle: urbanism, modernity and capital.

In searching for the (non)representation of epidemic disease within and between these forms of spectacle, I argue that principles of public health were often blocked and occasionally actively undermined by spectacular aesthetic investments in the city. Regimes of representation distorted by urban spectacle created an irregular and uneven vision of the city, characterised in practice less by the powerful *vue d'ensemble* or view from above, but by stymied forms of vision structured around spaces of ignorance and lapses in control.

## Plague in Morocco

Rabat and Casablanca were a showcase for a French urbanism built around the hygienic management of space and populations, and an architectural dream of clean lines, planned space, and gleaming surfaces. The outbreak and subsequent imbrication of plague and other infectious diseases in the Villes Modernes of Rabat and Casablanca, therefore, posed a particularly acute challenge to colonial ideologies of race, hygiene and hierarchy in North Africa. This stubborn, syncopated, episodic presence of plague in the modern cities and its insinuation into racially mixed working-class neighbourhoods did not jibe with colonial ideologies and imaginaries of the urban environment. Plague challenged the nascent science of urbanism which attempted to divide cities according to the given function of social space. Plague challenged serial narratives of modernisation and called for new theorisations of urban ecologies and the relationship of the city to its rural hinterland. Plague also challenged how far the demands of capital and heavy industry could be accommodated without stretching urban infrastructure too far and tipping the balance in favour of epidemics. The presence of plague in Rabat and Casablanca was both a colonial scandal – a secret that had to be suppressed – and an everyday planning heuristic that retraced and reshaped knowledge about the spaces and dispositions of the Moroccan body in the city.

Plague is believed to have been a constant presence throughout modern Moroccan history. The colonial doctor Raynaud estimated in 1902 that Morocco had suffered twenty-four epidemics of plague between 542 and 1818.[3] Medical authorities did not have a satisfactory explanation for the purported 'disappearance' of plague in the early nineteenth century, nor for its dramatic reappearance in Western Morocco in 1911–1912 in an epidemic that killed around 10,000 people. This outbreak had a significant impact on French doctors because it was a pneumonic form of plague with a correspondingly high mortality rate.[4] Writing in 1913 the doctor and Pasteurian Paul Remlinger described the re-emergence of plague as a set of separate and somewhat puzzling cases but argued that it should nonetheless be treated as the 'first manifestations of the twenty-fifth epidemic of plague in Morocco'.[5]

This 'twenty-fifth' epidemic had an epidemiological profile that resisted simple or linear interpretation. Outbreaks were likely to be unpredictable irruptions that affected single urban households or isolated rural villages. Rather than incubating in the countryside and spreading to the city as authorities expected it to, plague in Morocco appeared to be characterised by unpredictable exchanges between urban and rural populations. Was this one single distributed event or many isolated incidences? The peculiarities of Moroccan plague queried the rigid spatial boundaries imposed on Morocco by the French Protectorate and the corresponding strategic divisions in political authority.[6] The establishment of the French Protectorate was partly justified in terms of a French tutelage in biomedicine and public health and French hygienic texts, therefore, laid great emphasis on Morocco's unhygienic and chaotic past and its hygienic future. French authorities had a good reason, then, for locating plague outside of their purview. Writing in the 1930s, the colonial doctor Jules Colombani wrote: Plague has not reappeared in its epidemic form apart from the southern regions, in the unpacified territory. The few scattered outbreaks observed have remained geographically limited and besides have been quickly suppressed thanks to the efficacious measures put in place.[7]

The triumphalist note sounded in this text is, however, misleading, and its account of plague in the 1920s is partial. That there were no more epidemic outbreaks characterised by high mortality after 1911 did not imply that plague was no longer a significant matter of concern for colonial authorities. Colombani also failed to mention that the foyers of plague were either urban, emerging at the heart of the city, or close enough to the perimeter of the cities to suggest a characteristically suburban plague problem.

The presence of plague in the new cities of the Moroccan Protectorate thus presented an intellectual problem to be unpicked by the colonial sanitary authorities. Nowhere was this presence more puzzling than in the coastal cities of Rabat and Casablanca, cities that were the site of experiments in the planned management of social and sanitary space. Colonial authorities saw Rabat and Casablanca as a kind of urban 'frontier' presaging and shaping a future Moroccan nation-state.[8]

Rabat was the imperial capital, drawing upon the city's history for continuity with pre-colonial authority while creating 'an impressive modern setting for political control'.[9] Casablanca, an almost entirely European creation around a newly dug harbour, was planned as the financial and industrial centre.[10] A private sanitary report written in the early 1930s reflected that since 1911: 'there has barely been one year in which we have not registered some manifestation, large or small, of plague in the South or West of Morocco, and even in the cities Casablanca, Rabat, Sale and Kenitra'.[11] In 1917 a colonial doctor commented in a private report on the striking vulnerability of the new cities: 'Rabat, city of gardens, is the only city of the empire unable to rid itself of plague'.[12] In Rabat and Casablanca plague 'challenged the technocratic modernity of the new French colonial cities and illustrated the constructedness of white European settlers as 'civilised' and 'modern' populations'.[13]

## Figuring disease within scientific urbanism

The paradigmatic visual inscription of Rabat is the 'Plan Prost' – the schema created by the celebrated French urbanist to re-draw the city around culturally distinct and intelligible quarters: the Medina, the Mellah, and the Ville Nouvelle which was separated by a cordon sanitaire. These *quartiers* were aesthetically distinct with the Ville Nouvelle bisected by wide, tree-lined, Haussmanesque boulevards and striking architecture, and the Medina 'preserved' entirely as a 'monument' and 'shining vestige' of an ancient culture'.[14] The Ville Nouvelle of Rabat was built out and alongside a triangle formed by three cardinal points of Moroccan social and symbolic life. Sandwiched between and looped around by a no-build zone forming a cordon sanitaire was the Ville Nouvelle, characterised by its elegant public gardens and its Beaux-Arts public buildings and residential areas of villas.[15]

The 'view from above', the angle from which Moroccan cities were often conceptualised, drawn, and photographed, was a tool for the *aménagement du territoire*, the planned management of space. The aerial view of the city is an image and an inscription which, as de Certeau argues, corresponds most closely to the 'concept city', an entity which is characterised by the production of its own space and institutes itself as an autonomous political unit abstracted from larger social, political, and geographical spaces in which it is embedded.[16] The *aménagement du territoire* is best described as a particular technique of defining and directing the relationship between given territory, planned space, and social life. *Aménagement* seeks the best accommodations between nature, manufactured and material aspects of dwelling, such as architecture and infrastructure, and the symbolic conditions of living.[17] The deliberate coordination of these policies under the title of *aménagement* amounted, according to Henri Lefebvre, to the intentional production of space, the self-conscious 'spatialisation' of government.[18]

The Plan Prost was extensively visualised and exhibited, considered a spectacular achievement and an object of considerable intellectual and aesthetic interest. It was displayed prominently in the city and there is a proliferation of a sub-genre of photography, which positions Moroccans next to the displayed image of the splayed city. Where the city stands for the modern and technocratic pretensions of early twentieth century urbanists in much of the literature on Moroccan cities, it circulated through a range of visual iterations. In an image composed by the cinematographer and photographer Gabriel Veyre, we see the Plan Prost appear not as an abstracted inscription indicating or otherwise representing the idealised city, but as part of a collage of images representing distributed authority. These images represent French colonial power; the main part of the image shows General Lyautey inspecting a plan, the Plan Prost exposed in the background of the image. They are annotated by images displayed alongside, which portray colonial power operating in tandem with Alawid authority, a depiction of syncretic colonial culture.

The Plan Prost also appears repeatedly in the archives, reproduced and discussed extensively in debates about how sanitary policy can be integrated into urban planning and whether the aims of urbanism are desirable or effective from a hygienist perspective. Hygiene certainly figured in the urbanists' training and prominently in their polemic, but public health authorities worried that this was little more than an aesthetic concern for high sheen surfaces and spatial segregation. The more arcane kinds of knowledge that revealed the distribution of disease across space: the flight path of malarial mosquitoes, the habits of rats, the capacity of disease vectors to subvert planned space, these questions were often overlooked by urbanists. Sanitary indiscipline was not confined to the slum but was also evident in wealthy residential areas where health inspectors bemoaned the 'vanity' of French settlers, who cultivated aromatic gardens and even dug ornamental ponds, which attracted malarial mosquitoes in numbers even higher than the improvised nearby slums. Influential French urbanists argued strongly that the 'chill' of the Villes Nouvelles, where 'concrete is king', should be tempered by a more authentically 'Moroccan' aesthetic indiscipline of the makeshift, haphazard, and the tumbledown, an attitude that the colonial geographer Augustin Bernard found infuriatingly complacent, reminding his readers that 'we have not come to Morocco only to create literature, to restore mosques and to entice tourists, we are also here to eradicate disease'.[19]

When plague broke out in Rabat in 1914 it was the impoverished Spanish construction workers brought to the city to build, and who were themselves living in improvised and derelict buildings inside and outside the Medina, who died. Ellen Amster shows that this outbreak required a discursive and visual re-framing of poor white bodies as racialised and as equivalent to Moroccan bodies.[20] These arguments were also reasoned spatially. French doctors noted of this plague outbreak that although Moroccans seemed to be uniquely susceptible to typhus; plague appeared to be a problem of parasites, of being *parasité* or infested with fleas and lice, and it therefore 'went without saying that the European of a lowly condition who has the same lifestyle as that of a poor native, runs, as a result exactly the same risks as that native'.[21] An urbanist discourse combined with what Andrew Apter terms the 'camera obscura of class' produced an analysis in which shared space and class identities suspended privileges that might be conferred by race.[22]

In Morocco, this expansion of the power of unhygienic space to infest bodies and define them as backward and contagious was most visible in the expansion of *aménagement* in its colonial applications to become a technique for intervening upon the body in its most concrete and intimate spaces. In the management of epidemics, *aménagement* became a capacious set of practices that set out to redefine and to intervene upon relations between urban space and bodies. As well as picturing, forming, and re-forming the relationships of separate zones of the city to one another, depicting the way that the city enfolded collectivities of bodies, *aménagement* became a technique of investigating and controlling Moroccan bodies and Moroccan homes. In sanitary reports, the *aménagement* of the urban body indicated the passage of Moroccan bodies through the de-lousing stations located on the perimeter of the 'European' cities. This passage had a pragmatic hygienic function, but colonial officials were not insensible to its symbolic and highly visual aspect. The spectacle of delousing on the threshold of the city was partly designed to instruct. Colombani expressed this policy in the following terms, positioning a variegated indigenous public as the audience for carefully constructed colonial sanitation spectacles:

> the education of the indigenous public is achieved through conferences, which target the literate population, including pupils and former pupils of the *Colleges Musulmanes*, and by visits to notables led by hygienists, and by the urban prophylactic infrastructure (delousing and disinfection stations, the burning of public waste, adding bleach to drinking water, etc.).[23]

Infrastructural interventions targeting the poorest and least desirable in Moroccan society sought a wide public as both public health measure and visual spectacle.

Moroccans were theorised by colonial geographers, sociologists, and ethnologists as engaging and producing private domestic space away from the gaze of the colonisers according to their own social and spiritual inclinations. *Aménagement* was also used to capture this habit and to refer to cultural forms of privacy, the ways in which Moroccans occupy their houses. This analytic was in turn employed to justify spatial segregation along aesthetic lines. As Bernard wrote:

> the *aménagement* of the urban house responds to a double need: in the first instance to hide from passers-by and even from visitors, the intimacy of the master of the house and in particular that of his women; in the second instance, this *aménagement* is designed to exclude heat, sun and dust. The house has no façade or opening onto the street; it can never be too ugly, too poor, too misshapen on the outside, nor can it be too delicious inside.[24]

Hygienists agreed that the penetration of the Moroccan dwelling and its ultimate reorganisation was necessary from an intellectual and from a public health perspective.

The political, economic, and religious order of the Medina, they argued, was the order which was 'inherent in the nature, in the very form of the house, and it will require a veritable revolution in Moroccan dwelling to achieve satisfactory [public health] outcomes'.[25] *Aménagement*, then, was not merely an urban planning technique embedded in maps and schemas, it implied also the production of structured material interventions capable of arranging, enfolding, and expelling bodies from cities. Rather than prefiguring the intensely abstract theorisation of French territorial planning of the late twentieth century, French urban *aménagement* in Rabat and Casablanca was more closely related to a French urban order which Paul Rabinow dates from the fifteenth century; an order 'conceived in terms of three elements – the house, the street, and the city – and the problem of how (legally, aesthetically, financially, socially, politically, and medically) to relate them'.[26]

## Urban coexistence and Moroccan modernities

In 1915 an exhibition the Franco-Moroccan exhibition was held in Casablanca. This exhibition certainly partook in the interrogation of urban space through the exposure of maps, plans, and the tools of nascent urban planning. What was of particular interest to the organisers of the exhibition, however, were the ways in which Moroccans visiting the space interacted with its quiddities.[27] The French scrutinised the Moroccan visitors, watching them move from *vitrine* to *vitrine*, speculating about what they might be seeing. How did they understand the way that the exhibition space scrunched and compressed the territory? Were the correspondences and associations traced between the commodities on display and the ethnic particularities these commodities evoked, transparent and comprehensible to them? They carefully reported the impressions of trusted Moroccan interlocutors, while complaining that 'the Arab does not open up to us'.[28] While the *sentiments profonds* of the estimated 120,000 Moroccan visitors remained obscure, they did glean some insight into how the space of the *foire* was experienced and interpreted.

The report that was written with the aim of evaluating the success and the impact of the exhibition expanded upon these observations made by the French of the Moroccans who visited. Firstly, they found the presence of Moroccans distinctly picturesque. They commented on the ease with which Moroccans inserted themselves and accommodated themselves within the exhibition space, reminiscent of an orientalist 'scene'. One French spectator commented approvingly that he had seen in the Meknes Pavillion, stretched out on a carpet, just as at ease as she might have been in her *gourbi*, a 'peasant' (*femme de fellah*) breastfeeding her baby.[29]

The Casablanca exhibition did not partake in the exhaustive panoptic or aesthetic objectives discussed, for example, by scholars such as Timothy Mitchell in relation to the Orientalist fairs.[30] The report ultimately concluded that the exhibition had been a failure: in the final account the Resident General described it as a '*un chai, un timide chai*' (a timid storehouse) lamenting that North African visitors had seen a shabby, petty, commercial visage of European colonialism, more concerned with labelling, exporting, and consuming than with a large-scale transformation of society. These colonial spectacles, however, failed and anxious, nonetheless how urban planners and inter-disciplinary theorists of the city spoke an evolving language of colonial spectacle, concerned with questions of privacy, sincerity, and access to the inner lives of Moroccans as well as questions about how those subjects might engage in the production of urban space.

The *aménagement* of Rabat asserts the symbolic subdivisions of space into racialised, segregated spaces with the antique Medina and its residents encircled by the Ville Nouvelle. However, the city was marked by constant transgressions of these boundaries and Moroccan inhabitants displayed an ease at moving between spaces that was considerably less picturesque when transported from the exhibition space and applied to the real city. Unwilling to stay in the quickly overcrowded Medina, Moroccans migrating from elsewhere created makeshift 'derbs' which the French were quick to label slums and shantytowns and to subject to constant surveillance and invasive hygienic measures such as de-insectisation.

On their journey towards urban citizenship and the promise of cultural and racial progress implied by the journey from the 'dirty' countryside to the 'healthy' city, the presence of Moroccans 'out of place' was difficult to manage. This trajectory was complicated by spatial and temporal coexistence, which was critiqued and satirised in the serial language of modernisation theory. As the urbanist and hygienist Michel Gaud wrote, 'While the replacement of the tent with the house is undoubtedly progress, the same cannot be said for the replacement of the tent with a *gourbi*' (an urban shack thought to be a very virulent and dangerous environment).[31] One newspaper editorial from 1932 argued that the French in Rabat had thus far not succeeded in critical projects of modernisation embedded in urban *aménagement*; they had not manufactured a new set of relations out of the materialities of territories, cities, and bodies, but in fact only succeeded in 'exporting' the *bidonville* (shantytown). In other words, the dirty, noisy, and smelly shantytown was a product of modernity and not an irruption of incongruous and antique ways of life in the heart of the city: 'if only the Protectorate had assisted the unfortunates to construct houses which were both hygienic and aesthetic (as these are the two preoccupations of our Moroccan brothers), the slums of Douar el Doum would not exist'.[32]

### *Terrains vagues:* capital, control, and the recuperation of space in Casablanca

In contrast to the curatorial duties that weighed upon city planners in Rabat and sketched in the lines of the Plan Prost, Casablanca was considered lucky ('*heureuse*') to have no existing Medina whose aesthetic had to be preserved or curated by city planners.[33] Less concerned with aesthetic unity and more with serving the city's commercial interests, Henri Prost's plan for Casablanca 'vertebrated' the city with four large intersecting arteries that would bring in grain from the regions to be processed and exported.[34] Casablanca was, however, unluckily located, in that it was embedded in a region well known for its unsanitary countryside and in particular for its endemic foyers of plague.[35] Perceived by sanitary authorities as being hemmed around by a hostile and unhygienic rural proletariat eager to enter the city, Casablanca thus required a particular form of urban management. A dedicated sub-regional hygiene and public health service was established which separated Casablanca from the region. This decision was justified through a reference to the exceptional qualities of Casablanca and its particular vulnerability to disease. Any epidemic breaking out in Casablanca would have to be dealt with promptly because of the commercial interest in keeping the port city free of disease. Moreover, Casablanca provided 'propitious terrain' for epidemics because it was 'a city under construction'. This status also necessitated a particular approach, because 'the ordinary toolkit of a city already completely constituted is not suitable for this city characterised by huge movement and upheaval'.[36] The image of a city under construction was taken up satirically by an editorial in Le Petit Marocain in 1932 which suggested that Casablanca was a failed city characterised not by the picturesque ruins of Rabat but by its own *ruines officielles*.[37]

The idea of Casablanca as a city under formation, in the process of construction, and therefore permeable and vulnerable to convulsions, failures of planning, and epidemics, was central not only to scientific urbanism but to the urban sensorium of the two cities. The characteristics of the city, its kinetic energy and its distinctive unfinished shoddiness, were evoked in sentimental tributes to its seedy charm and indicted by sanitary officers and urban theorists. Hygienists Gaud and Bonjean writing in 1937 drew a sobering comparison between Fez *compartimentée dans ces antiques murailles* and Casablanca's fundamental troubling 'openness'. This had resulted in the city turned inside out and resulted in the entanglement (*l'intrication*) of the *derbs* within the city.[38] Where Rabat was understood through the prism of serial modernities, Casablanca with its fast and unchecked growth folded the rural and suburban into its urban fabric.

In Casablanca, rampant land speculation led to chaotic and unplanned construction which carved out '*terrain vagues*' of unplanned and unenclosed space.[39] The *terrains vagues* were legal and sanitary blanks on the maps and opened up the heart of the city to rural Moroccans who used them opportunistically to construct temporary dwellings. Both Henri Prost and later the architect and urbanist Michel Ecochard argued that Moroccan workers' houses should be built around enclosed space.[40] Indeed, Ecochard's plan for Casablanca proposed to deploy the *trame sanitaire* with its living space around an encircled 'arabic patio'. A reading of the archives, however, evince a palpable fear of mixing Moroccans and open spaces, of leaving space, public or private, which people can dispose of and create themselves. This fear, expressed in private correspondence characterised by a laconic, pragmatic, anti-aesthetic, and rather anti-intellectual attitude, often accused the Protectorate's architects of 'fictitious' planning (an observation that blended the insinuation of commercial speculation with the allegation of unrealistic or at least overly theoretical planning). To the construction of a *cité ouvrier* in Casablanca in 1921, one official expressed his opinion that the generous allocation of '*espaces verts*', green leisure space bordering and adjoining the workers' housing, was unreasonable:

it should be clear to you that these constructions will be occupied for the most part by workers, who will have neither the time nor the means to take care of over 200 square metres of gardens and that these open spaces will be quickly transformed into a dumping ground for any imaginable object and will become open-air laundries in no time . . . this will perhaps be considered picturesque in the eye of certain artists, but it will quickly make the new *quartier* into a foyer of infection and of epidemics . . . these observations are based on the evidence that we see every day in Morocco's Ville Nouvelle*s*, especially in areas occupied by the working classes.[41]

The failure of Casablanca's *aménagement* would seem to have been a failure to adequately and wholly grasp the city as an ensemble; a failure to take into account in planning terms the view from above. In Casablanca, however, another form of vision ran counter to the bird's eye view: the desire to create a kind of monumental space bisected by lateral 'views'. Whereas in Rabat the imagined citizen might stroll along the walls of the Medina consuming and admiring the view, in Casablanca the imagined citizen should take in the 'perspectives' offered by the wide, flat boulevards that offered a directed perspective and an untrammelled gaze. The ideal of the extension of vision across space was quickly broken by rapid building and land speculation, in 1932 the socialist newspaper *La Vigie Marocaine* protested in a newspaper editorial that what passed for a 'public plan of the city' in Casablanca (the city's equivalent of the Plan Prost) was 'in actual fact the preparation of a vast building plot' (*un vaste lotissement*). The 'good' bourgeois *colons* who had followed the rules and invested in villas in new *quartiers* as Casablanca extended outwards into its rural hinterland now found themselves 'hemmed in', their view broken by the extravagant billboards that surrounded their houses.[42]

As well as raising the spectre of the commercial and unhygienic recuperation of space, the *terrains vagues* threw the identity and integrity of particular spaces into question. *Terrains vagues* were particularly focused around the empty spaces surrounding the new roads and in the indeterminate zone of the suburban, where new workers' housing pushed up against slums, and slums shaded dangerously into the countryside. When plague broke out in Casablanca in 1945, it struck Europeans and Moroccans and was focused around the grain silos located at the centre of the city and perilously close to the harbour. In 1946 a doctor at the Moroccan Institute of Hygiene noted that over the course of this epidemic Casablanca's great wide roads, built to channel goods out of the country had become 'veritable avenues of plague'.[43] One urban granary worker was even thought to be responsible for carrying plague out of the city and infecting a household in the rural hinterland – reversing the direction in which contagion and contagious subjects were assumed to flow. This reversal made plague uniquely challenging as an epidemic event, as a textured experience of the urban everyday embedded in highly mediatised rituals of sanitation, as an open secret, and – as I have argued – as a kind of heuristic for various forms of planning strategies.

## Conclusion

More than any other contagious disease, plague in Morocco dissolved boundaries between the Medina and the Ville Nouvelle necessitating a granular social optics of class to analyse the causes of disease and reversing ecological assumptions about the modern city and its relation to its rural hinterland. Just as the intimate colonial ethnology of the Moroccan home and modes of dwelling in the modern city emphasised its 'reversed' *aménagement*, its inversion of the modernist aesthetic ideal of the urban civility, in which good citizenship entails presenting a best aspect outwards towards the city: plague turned the colonial city inside out. The presence of plague presented a challenge to the technocratic modernity of the planned city and led people to question the promise of better health embedded in urbanist technique. Public health authorities struggled with the reality that urbanisation, modernisation, and the penetration of capital had no protective capacities against epidemic disease; indeed, they frequently exposed city dwellers to new forms of complex and unpredictable risk.

## Notes

1 Research leading to this chapter was funded by the European Research Council Starting Grant under the European Union's Seventh Framework Programme/ERC grant agreement no. 336564; European Research Council [FP7/2007–2013] for the projectVisual Representations of theThird Plague Pandemic (CRASSH, University of Cambridge).
2 Wald, *Contagious.*
3 Raynaud, *Etude sur l'hygiène.*
4 Martinez-Antonio, 'L'année de la peste'.
5 Remlinger, 'La Peste au Maroc', 12.
6 The French Protectorate in Morocco was established in 1912 via the Treaty of Fes. The Treaty defined the French *makhzan* policy, preserving the Moroccan monarchy while exercising indirect rule. While ostensibly governing with and alongside the Alawid Sultan, French colonialism in Morocco fundamentally changed the organisation and political status of Moroccan territory while framing the French role as that of paternalistic 'protector' overseeing a process of modernisation. Pre-Protectorate Morocco was believed to be divided into two fundamentally antagonistic elements; the *bled el-makhzan*, territory governed by the central government or *Makhzan*, and the *bled el-siba*, territory characterised by nomadism and resistance to the *Makhzan*. French administrators drew upon ethnological and sociological knowledge to claim that the *makhzan* was 'failed', as it had not succeeded in making Morocco an integrated and legible territory; see Sebti, 'Colonial Experience and Territorial Practices'; Burke III, *The Ethnographic State.*
7 Colombani, *La Protection Sanitaire*, 5–6.
8 Wright, *The Politics of Design*, 92.
9 *Ibid.*
10 Rabat and Casablanca were linked to one another via their aesthetic intentions although they were perceived as having evolved along divergent paths. From the vantage point of Rabat egregious and dysfunctional developments in planning often raised the spectre of become 'as bad as Casablanca'. In postcolonial Morocco the cities retain distinct characteristics in the eyes of urbanised Moroccans while for rural populations Rabat and Casablanca form part of a 'single urban agglomeration', Ossman, *Picturing Casablanca*, 29.

11 'La Prophylaxie de la Peste au Maroc' (Archives du Maroc, Box Number E850).

12 Amster, *Medicine and the Saints*, 127.

13 *Ibid.*, 111.

14 Rabinow, *French Modern*, 300.

15 The Plan Prost already contained, however, a pragmatic accommodation with the material reality of the city. As European speculators had pre-empted the planned city by building working class neighbourhoods abutting the Medina, the hygienic separation between old and new building was already made incoherent. Prost therefore enclosed the Medina with boulevards which had the dual aesthetic advantages of encoding Haussman's association of wide boulevards with space, light and circulation and providing a place in the city from which to linger and admire the ancient walls of the old town. Haussman's urban values are transformed here into techniques of racial segregation and tools for shaping the gaze of urban citizens. See Amster, *Medicine and the Saints.*

16 de Certeau, *The Practice of Everyday Life.*

17 For an account of the history of the technique in France see Wendeln, *Contested Territory*; Desportes and Picon, *De l'Espace au Territoire.*

18 Wendeln, *Contested Territory.*

19 Bernard, *L'habitation Indigène.*

20 Amster, *Medicine and the Saints.*

21 'La Prophylaxie de la Peste au Maroc' (BGR, Box number E850), 3, see also Jorge, *A Propos de la Peste au Maroc.*

22 Apter, *Beyond Words*, 142.

23 Columbani, *La Protection Sanitaire*, 6

24 Bernard, *L'habitation Indigène*, 18.

25 Gaud and Sicault, 'L'habitat Indigène', 58.

26 Rabinow, *French Modern*, 74.

27 That this was a distinctively commercial event intended to showcase the commodities that could be collected and monetised from the French North African colony and protectorates indicates an early commodification of urban space.

28 Exposition Franco-Marocaine, *Rapport Général et Rapports des Sections* (Casablanca, 1919), 48.

29 Exposition Franco-Marocaine, *Rapport Général et Rapports des Sections* (Casablanca, 1919).

30 Mitchell, *Colonising Egypt.*

31 Bernard, *L'habitation Indigène*, 18.

32 Archives du Maroc (Box S265).

33 'The respect for the artistic and social integrity of the old Medinas does not apply to Casablanca, luckily without monuments and without a past', Marrast, *L'Oeuvre d'Henri Prost*, 61.

34 Haffner, *The View from Above*, 96.

35 Gaud, 'Epidemie de peste'.

36 Extrait de Bulletin Officiel no. 85 19 Juin 1914, 459 'Decision residentielle sur l'hygiène et l'assistance publiques a Casablanca' (Archives du Maroc, Box Number E4504).

37 *Petit Marocain*, 11 February 1932.

38 Gaud and Bonjean, 'Considerations sur l'epidemiologie', 23–25.

39 Janet Abu-Lughod describes the same process in Rabat in the following terms: 'At all weak points in the urban fabric the pressures of Moroccan needs for space had broken through, resulting in enclaves, some large, such as Dabbagh and Doum, most small and uncaptured by the statistics – that were beginning to give the original neatly bifurcated urban design a checkerboard appearance' Abu-Lughod, *Rabat*, 221.

40 Ecochard, *Casablanca.*

41 Habitations à bon marché (Archives du Maroc, Box A1414).

42 *La Vigie Marocaine*, 29 June 1932.

43 Quoted in Gaud, 'Epidemie de peste', 39.

# References

Abu-Lughod, Janet L., *Rabat: Urban Apartheid in Morocco* (Princeton: Princeton University Press, 1980).

Amster, Ellen, *Medicine and the Saints: Science, Islam and the Colonial Encounter in Morocco, 1877–1956* (Austin: University of Texas Press, 2014).

Apter, Andrew, *Beyond Words: Discourse and Critical Agency in Africa* (Chicago: University of Chicago Press, 2007).

Apter, Andrew, 'On Imperial Spectacle: The Dialectics of Seeing in Colonial Nigeria', *Comparative Studies in Society and History*, 44, 3 (2002), 564–596.

Bernard, Augustin, *L'habitation Indigène dans les Possessions Françaises* (Paris-Vanves: impr. Kapp, Paris, 1932).

Bigon, Liora, 'Bubonic Plague, Colonial Ideologies, and Urban Planning Policies: Dakar, Lagos, and Kumasi', *Planning Perspectives*, 31, 2 (2016), 205–226.

Burke III, Edmund, *The Ethnographic State: France and the Invention of Moroccan Islam* (California: University of California Press, 2014).

de Certeau, Michel, *The Practice of Everyday Life* (Berkeley: University of California Press, 1984).

Colombani, Jules, *La Protection Sanitaire de l'Indigène au Maroc* (Paris: H. Blanc and G. Gautier, 1932).

Dawdy, Shannon Lee, 'Profane Archaeology and the Existential Dialectics of the City', *Journal of Social Archeology*, 16, 1 (2016), 32–55.

Desportes, Marc and Antoine Picon, *De l'Espace au Territoire: L'amenagement en France (16e-20e siècles)* (Paris: Presses de l'ENPC, 1997).

Ecochard, Michel, *Casablanca: Le roman d'une ville* (Paris: Ed. de Paris, 1955).

Gaud, Michel, 'Epidemie de peste de la Chaouia', *Bulletin de l'Institut d'Hygiène de Maroc*, 1 (1945), 31–49.

Gaud, Michel and Claude Bonjean, 'Considerations sur l'epidemiologie du typhus dans l'Afrique du Nord', *Bulletin de l'Hygiène de Maroc*, 2–3 (1937), 23–45.

Gaud, Michel and Georges Sicault, 'L'habitat Indigène au Maroc', *Bulletin de l'Hygiène du Maroc*, 4 (1937).

Haffner, Jeanne, *The View from Above: The Science of Social Space* (Cambridge, MA: MIT Press, 2013).

Jorge, Ricardo, 'A propos de la peste au Maroc et de la leçon de prophlyaxie qui s'en dégage', *Bulletin de l'Hygiène de Maroc*, 2–3 (1932), 34–48.

Marrast, Jean, *L'Oeuvre d'Henri Prost: Architecture et Urbanisme* (Paris: Académie d'Architecture, 1960).

Martinez-Antonio, Francisco Javier, 'L'année de la peste: santé publique et impérialism français au Maroc autour de la crise d'Agadir', *Mélanges de la Casa de Velazquez*, 44, 1 (2014), 251–273.

Mitchell, Timothy, *Colonising Egypt* (Berkeley: University of California Press, 1988).

Myers, Garth Andrew, *Verandahs of Power: Colonialism and Space in Urban Africa* (New York: Syracuse University Press, 2003).

Ossman, Susan, *Picturing Casablanca: Portrait of Power in a Modern City* (Berkeley: University of California Press, 1994).

Otter, Chris, 'Making Liberalism Durable: Vision and Civility in the late Victorian City', *Social History*, 27, 1 (2002), 1–15.

Rabinow, Paul, *French Modern: Norms and Forms of the Social Environment* (Chicago: University of Chicago Press, 1995).

Raynaud, L., *Etude sur l'hygiène et la medicine au Maroc* (Paris: Alger, 1902).

Remlinger, Paul, 'La Peste au Maroc', *Revue d'hygiène et de police sanitaire*, 35 (1913), 11–24.

Sebti, Abdelahad, 'Colonial Experience and Territorial Practices', in: Driss Maghraoui (ed.), *Revisiting the Colonial Past in Morocco* (London and New York: Routledge, 2013), 38–56.

Swanson, Maynard, 'The Sanitation Syndrome: Bubonic Plague and Urban Native Policy in the Cape Colony, 1900–1909', *The Journal of African History*, 18, 3 (1977), 387–410.

Wald, Priscilla, *Contagious: Cultures, Carriers, and the Outbreak Narrative* (Durham, NC: Duke University Press, 2007).

Wendeln, Matthew, 'Contested Territory: Regional Development in France, 1934–1968' (PhD Dissertation, New York University, 2011).

Wright, Gwendolyn, *The Politics of Design in French Colonial Urbanism* (Chicago: University of Chicago Press, 1992).

# INDEX